Interpreting Laboratory Data

A Point-of-Care Guide

Justin Schmidt, PharmD, BCPS

Assistant Professor
Midwestern University
Chicago College of Pharmacy
Downers Grove, Illinois

Jeffrey Wieczorkiewicz, PharmD, BCPS

Assistant Professor
Midwestern University
Chicago College of Pharmacy
Downers Grove, Illinois

American Society of Health-System Pharmacists®

Bethesda, Maryland

Any correspondence regarding this publication should be sent to the publisher, American Society of Health-System Pharmacists, 7272 Wisconsin Avenue, Bethesda, MD 20814, attention: Special Publishing.

The information presented herein reflects the opinions of the contributors and advisors. It should not be interpreted as an official policy of ASHP or as an endorsement of any product.

Because of ongoing research and improvements in technology, the information and its applications contained in this text are constantly evolving and are subject to the professional judgment and interpretation of the practitioner due to the uniqueness of a clinical situation. The editors, contributors, and ASHP have made reasonable efforts to ensure the accuracy and appropriateness of the information presented in this document. However, any user of this information is advised that the editors, contributors, advisors, and ASHP are not responsible for the continued currency of the information, for any errors or omissions, and/or for any consequences arising from the use of the information in the document in any and all practice settings. Any reader of this document is cautioned that ASHP makes no representation, guarantee, or warranty, express or implied, as to the accuracy and appropriateness of the information contained in this document and specifically disclaims any liability to any party for the accuracy and/or completeness of the material or for any damages arising out of the use or non-use of any of the information contained in this document.

Director, Special Publishing: Jack Bruggeman
Acquisitions Editor: Jack Bruggeman
Senior Editorial Project Manager: Dana Battaglia
Production Editor: Kristin Eckles
Design: David Wade

ISBN 978-1-58528-263-0

DEDICATION

I would like to thank my lovely wife, Valerie, for her support and instrumental help reviewing this book and my family for their support.

Justin

I would like to thank my beautiful wife, Sarah, and my two wonderful daughters, Madelyn and Francesca, for all of their support. I would also like to thank my family for their continued support.

Jeffrey

ACKNOWLEDGMENTS

We would like to acknowledge the original contributors, reviewers, and Mary Lee, PharmD, BCPS, FCCP, editor of *Basic Skills in Interpreting Laboratory Data* for creating and shaping much of the content in this reference. We would also like to thank Nancy Fjortoft, PhD and Sue Winkler, PharmD, BCPS, our Dean and Department Chair respectively, for providing us the opportunity to work on this project and Julie Stein-Gocken, PharmD for providing support at our clinical site. We also owe gratitude to Dana Battaglia, Sr. editorial project manager, Jack Bruggeman, special publishing director, and the ASHP Special Publications group, which provided guidance and valuable input into the design and construction of this reference.

Justin and Jeffrey

Contributors to *Basic Skills in Interpreting Laboratory Data, Fourth Edition*

Sheila M. Allen, PharmD, BCPS

Kendra M. Atkinson, PharmD

Amber L. Beitelshees, PharmD, MPH

Jill S. Borchert, PharmD, BCPS

Candace S. Brown, MSN, PharmD, BPS
   Certified in Psychopharmacy

Lingtak-Neander Chan, PharmD, BCNSP

Peter A. Chyka, PharmD, DABAT,
   FAACT

Samir Y. Dahdal, MD, FACC

Wafa Y. Dahdal, PharmD, BCPS
   (AQ Cardiology)

Lea E. dela Peña, PharmD, BCPS

Philip F. Dupont, MD, PhD

Sharon M. Erdman, PharmD

Joshua D. Farkas, MD, MS

Paul Farkas, MD

Edward F. Foote, PharmD, FCCP, BCPS

Thomas G. Hall, PharmD, BCPS, FASHP

Paul R. Hutson, PharmD, BCOP

Min J. Joo, MD, MPH

Donna M. Kraus, PharmD

Alan Lau, PharmD

Mary Lee, PharmD, BCPS, FCCP

Frank W. Ling, MD

Janis J. MacKichan, PharmD, FAPhA

Robb McGory, MS, PharmD

Patrick J. Medina, PharmD, BCOP

Keith A. Rodvold, PharmD, FCCP, FIDSA

Terry L. Schwinghammer, PharmD,
   FCCP, FASHP, BCPS

Roohollah Sharifi, MD, FACS

Karen J. Tietze, PharmD

Dominick P. Trombetta, PharmD, BCPS, CGP, FASCP

Eva M. Vivian, PharmD, BCPS, CDE, BC-ADM

Lori A. Wilken, PharmD, TT-S, AE-C, CDE

Issam Zineh, PharmD, MPH

Content Reviewer for *Interpreting Laboratory Data: A Point-of-Care Guide*

Ambra King, PharmD
Medication Use Safety Specialty Resident
The Johns Hopkins Hospital
Baltimore, Maryland

CONTENTS

PREFACE

In 2010, we received word that ASHP Special Publishing was interested in creating a point-of-care guide to accompany *Basic Skills in Interpreting Laboratory Data, 4th Edition*. The idea stemmed from market feedback that concluded a concise reference about interpreting laboratory values geared toward pharmacists would be beneficial. Feedback indicated that the use of quickview charts (concise laboratory monographs, which appear in the 4th edition to display pertinent laboratory data) would be a great start to a new reference (see sample chart). While other point-of-care references are available for interpretation of laboratory values, they are not generally focused on information most relevant to pharmacy students and pharmacists. Often, information is extraneous or incomplete from the pharmacist's perspective.

The goal of *Basic Skills in Interpreting Laboratory Data, 4th Edition,* is to provide information on common laboratory tests used to screen for or diagnose disease, monitor the effectiveness and safety of treatment, or assess disease severity for pharmacy students, pharmacy residents, and practicing pharmacists. Our aim is to provide a resource that provides concise information at the point-of-care about pertinent laboratory values and their corresponding assays. When abnormal laboratory values arise, it is important to determine the relevance and potential etiology. This pocket reference will facilitate interpretation of laboratory results and help evaluate potential relationships with medications and disease states. Once the laboratory results are appropriately evaluated, more informed decisions can be made regarding optimal pharmacotherapy and disease state management to improve patient outcomes.

While this book works as a companion to the parent text, it is designed to be used by residents and practitioners in their everyday practice. The bulk of the text comprises laboratory monographs arranged alphabetically. There was consideration for a topic-based approach as is present in the parent text, but the decision to arrange the charts alphabetically stemmed from the idea that the text would be most often utilized by pharmacists evaluating available laboratory results, and, therefore, an alphabetical listing would be more user-friendly. As pharmacists may not know the relevance of the laboratory result to a disease, an approach starting from the laboratory values was deemed the most logical. A topic index was created to allow for identification of laboratory values that might be appropriate based on disease states. Appendices were created to provide supplemental information about laboratory methods, collection, and statistical concepts related to diagnosis. When asked about the desired format, mixed feedback regarding the medium of content (paper vs. electronic) was provided. With this in mind, we worked with ASHP to ensure that the content would translate well to electronic formats.

Justin Schmidt
Jeffrey Wieczorkiewicz
September 2011

ABBREVIATIONS

Abbreviation	Expanded
μL	microliter
μmol	micromole
6-MP	6-mercaptopurine
ABG	arterial blood gas
ACEIs	angiotensin converting enzyme inhibitors
ACS	acute coronary syndrome
ACTH	adrenocorticotropic hormone
ADA	American Diabetic Association
ADEs	adverse drug events
ADH	antidiuretic hormone
ADRs	adverse drug reactions
aFp	alpha fetoprotein
AG	anion gap
AIDS	acquired immune deficiency syndrome
Al	aluminum
ALL	acute lymphoblastic leukemia
ALP	alkaline phosphatase
ALT	alanine aminotransferase
AML	acute myelogenous leukemia
ANA	antinuclear antibodies
APAP	acetyl-p-aminophenol (acetaminophen)
APC	activated protein C
aPTT	activated partial thromboplastin time
ARAs	aldosterone receptor antagonists
ARB	angiotensin receptor blocker

ASA	acetyl-salicylic acid (aspirin)
AST	aspartate aminotransferase
ATP	adenosine triphosphate
AUC	area under the curve
AV	atrioventricular
B2M	beta-2 microglobulin
BMI	body mass index
BNP	B-type natriuretic peptide
BP	blood pressure
BPH	benign prostatic hypertrophy
BUN	blood urea nitrogen
Ca	calcium
CA	cancer antigen
CAD	coronary artery disease
CEA	carcinoembryonic antigen
CHD	coronary heart disease
CHF	chronic heart failure
CK	creatine kinase
CKD	chronic kidney disease
Cl	chloride
CrCl	creatinine clearance
CML	chronic myelogenous leukemia
CMV	cytomegalovirus
CNS	central nervous system
CO_2	carbon dioxide
COPD	chronic obstructive pulmonary disease
Cr^{3+}	chromium
CRH	corticotropin releasing hormone

CSF	cerebrospinal fluid
CSNs	cephalosporins
CV	cardiovascular
CVA	cerebrovascular accident
DHEAS	dehydroepiandrosterone sulfate
DIC	disseminated intravascular coagulation
dL	deciliter
DM	diabetes mellitus
DNA	deoxyribonucleic acid
DPG	diphosphoglycerate
DVT	deep vein thrombosis
e.g.	for example
ECF	extracellular fluid
ECG	electrocardiogram
EKG	electrocardiogram
ELISA	enzyme linked immunosorbent assay
ESA	erythropoietin stimulating agent
FDA	Food and Drug Administration
FEV_1	forced expiratory volume in 1 second
FFP	fresh frozen plasma
FiO_2	fraction of inspired oxygen
FISH	fluorescence in situ hybridization
fL	femtoliter
FSH	follicle stimulating hormone
FVC	forced vital capacity
g	gram
G6PD	glucose 6 phosphate dehydrogenase
GABA	gamma aminobutyric acid

G-CSF	granulocyte colony stimulating factor
GFR	glomerular filtration rate
GGTP	gamma-glutamyl transpeptidase
GHRH	growth hormone releasing hormone
GI	gastrointestinal
GM-CSF	granulocyte-macrophage colony stimulating factor
GnRH	gonadotropin releasing hormone
GP2b3a	glycoprotein 2b3a
GU	genitourinary
HA	headache
HCl	hydrochloric acid
HCO_3	bicarbonate
Hct	hematocrit
HD	hemodialysis
HER-2	human epidermal growth factor receptor 2
Hgb	hemoglobin
HIT	heparin-induced thrombocytopenia
HIV	human immunodeficiency virus
HMG-COA	hydroxymethylglutaryl CoA
HPLC	high performance liquid chromatography
HR	heart rate
hr	hour
HTN	hypertension
IBD	inflammatory bowel disease
ICF	intracellular fluid
IDA	iron deficiency anemia
IHC	immunohistochemistry
IL-2	interleukin-2

IM	intramuscular
INR	international normalized ratio
ITP	idiopathic thrombocytopenic purpura
IU	international unit
IV	intravenous
K	potassium
L	liter
LDH	lactic acid dehydrogenase
LDL	low density lipoprotein
LH	luteinizing hormone
LMWH	low molecular weight heparin
LSD	lysergic acid diethylamide
MAOIs	monoamine oxidase inhibitors
mcg	microgram
MCH	mean corpuscular hemoglobin
MCHC	mean corpuscular hemoglobin concentration
MCTD	mixed connective tissue disease
MCV	mean corpuscular volume
mEq	milliequivalents
mg	milligram
Mg	magnesium
MHC	major histocompatibility complex
MI	myocardial infarction
min	minute
mL	milliliter
mm	millimeter
MMF	mycophenolate mofetil
mmHg	millimeters of mercury

mmol	millimole
mo	month
mOsm	milliosmole
mRNA	messenger ribonucleic acid
N/A	non-applicable or not available
N/V	nausea and vomiting
N/V/D	nausea, vomiting, and diarrhea
Na	sodium
NaHCO$_3$	sodium bicarbonate
NAPA	n-acetyl procainamide
ng	nanogram
nmol	nanomole
NSAID	nonsteroidal anti-inflammatory drugs
NT-proBNP	N terminal pro B-type natriuretic peptide
O$_2$	oxygen
OHP	hydroxyprogesterone
PaCO$_2$	partial pressure of arterial carbon dioxide
PaO$_2$	partial pressure of arterial oxygen
PCNs	penicillins
PCO$_2$	partial pressure of arterial carbon dioxide
PCOS	polycystic ovary syndrome
PCP	phencyclidine
PCR	polymerase chain reaction
PE	pulmonary embolism
PEFR	peak expiratory flow rate
PF4	platelet factor 4
pg	picogram
PGP	p-glycoprotein

PO_2	partial pressure of arterial oxygen
PPIs	proton pump inhibitors
PSA	prostate-specific antigen
PT	prothrombin time
PTT	partial thromboplastin time
PTU	propylthiouracil
RA	rheumatoid arthritis
RBC	red blood cell
RDW	red blood cell distribution width
RNA	ribonucleic acid
RTA	renal tubular acidosis
SCr	serum creatinine
sec	second
SHBG	sex hormone binding globulin
SIADH	syndrome of inappropriate antidiuretic hormone
SLE	systemic lupus erythematosus
SOB	shortness of breath
SRA	serotonin release assay
SSRIs	selective serotonin reuptake inhibitors
St	saint
sx	symptoms
TB	tuberculosis
TBG	thyroxine binding globulins
TCAs	tricyclic antidepressants
TCO_2	total carbon dioxide
TdP	torsades de pointes
TIBC	total iron binding capacity
TnI	troponin I

Tobra	tobramycin
TPMT	thiopurine methyltransferase
TPN	total parenteral nutrition
TSAT	transferrin saturation
TTP	thrombotic thrombocytopenic purpura
TZD	thiazide
UFH	unfractionated heparin
μL	microliter
ULN	upper limit of normal
US	United States
vit	vitamin
wk	week
yr	year

FORMAT AND CONTENT OF A QUICKVIEW CHART

TEST NAME		
PARAMETER	**DESCRIPTION**	**COMMENTS**
Common reference range		
Adults	Reference range in adults	Variability and factors affecting range
Pediatrics	Reference range in children	
Critical value	Value beyond which immediate action usually needs to be taken	Disease-dependent factors; relative to reference range; value is a multiple of upper normal limit
Inherent activity	Does substance have any physiological activity?	Description of activity and factors affecting activity
Location		
Production	Is substance produced? If so, where?	Factors affecting production
Storage	Is substance stored? If so, where?	Factors affecting storage
Secretion/ excretion	Is substance secreted /excreted? If so, where/how?	Factors affecting secretion or excretion
Causes of abnormal levels		
High	Major causes	Modification of circumstances, other related causes or drugs that are commonly monitored with this test
Low	Major causes	
Signs and symptoms		
High level	Major signs and symptoms with a high or positive result	Modification of circumstances/ other related signs and symptoms
Low level	Major signs and symptoms with a low or negative result	
After event, time to…		
Initial elevation	Minutes, hours, days, weeks	Assumes acute insult
Peak values	Minutes, hours, days, weeks	Assumes insult not yet removed
Normalization	Minutes, hours, days, weeks	Assumes insult removed and nonpermanent damage
Causes of spurious results	List of common causes	Modification of circumstances/ assay specific
Additional info	Any other pertinent information regarding the lab value or assay	

1→ 3 β-D-Glucan

PARAMETER	DESCRIPTION	COMMENTS
Common reference range	Negative	
Critical value	Positive	Highly immunogenic component released by the fungal cell wall
Inherent activity	None	
Location		
Production	Fungal cell wall	
Storage	Serum	
Secretion/ excretion	N/A	
Causes of abnormal levels		
High	Fungal infection	May suggest presence of a number of potential fungal pathogens including, but not limited to, *Aspergillus* sp., *Candida* sp., *Fusarium* sp., and *Trichosporon* sp.
Low	N/A	
Signs and symptoms		
High level	Related to underlying fungal infection	
Low level	N/A	
After event, time until…		
Initial elevation	N/A	
Peak values	N/A	
Normalization	N/A	
Causes of spurious results	N/A	
Additional info	Test is performed to use in conjunction with other diagnostic methods to support the diagnosis of invasive fungal infections	

Adrenocorticotropic Hormone (ACTH)

PARAMETER	DESCRIPTION	COMMENTS
Common reference range	5–10 mcg/dL	
Critical value	<5 mcg/dL	
	>10 mcg/dL	
Inherent activity	Yes	Stimulates cortisol production
Location		
Production	Anterior pituitary	
Secretion/excretion	N/A	
Causes of abnormal levels		
High	Pituitary tumor	
	ACTH secreting ectopic tumor	ACTH dependent
	Adrenal tumor	
Low	Corticosteroids	Levels not commonly monitored with listed medication
	Adrenal tumor	ACTH independent
Signs and symptoms		
High level	Facial plethora, fat accumulation, central obesity, hypertension, osteoporosis, depression, myopathies	
Low level	Weakness, weight loss, hypotension, postural dizziness, vertigo, gastrointestinal symptoms	
After event, time until...		
Initial elevation	N/A	
Peak values	N/A	
Normalization	N/A	
Causes of spurious results	N/A	
Additional info	Plasma ACTH and cortisol levels exhibit peaks (6–8 a.m.) and nadirs (11 p.m.)	

Alanine Aminotransferase (ALT)

PARAMETER	DESCRIPTION	COMMENTS
Common reference range		
Adults	3–30 International Units/L	Varies with assay
Newborns	3–60 International Units/L	Decreases to adult values within a few months
Critical value	>60 International Units/L	>2 times upper limit of normal
Inherent activity	Yes	Intracellular enzymatic activity
Location		
Production	Intracellular enzyme	
Storage	Liver, muscle, heart, kidney	These tissues are rich in ALT
Secretion/ excretion	None	
Causes of abnormal levels		
High	Isoniazid, HMG-COA inhibitors, allopurinol, methotrexate, ketoconazole, valproic acid	Listed medications are routinely monitored
	Hepatitis, hemolysis, muscular diseases, MI, renal infarction	Elevated in any disease with hepatocyte (liver cell) inflammation
		Elevated in any disease with damage to tissues rich in enzyme
Low	N/A	
Signs and symptoms		
High level	Varies with underlying disease	Reflects tissue or organ damage
Low level	N/A	
After event, time until…		
Initial elevation	2–6 hr	
Peak values	24–48 hr (without further cell damage)	With extensive liver or cellular damage, levels can go up to thousands
Normalization	24–48 hr	Assumes insult removed and no ongoing damage
Causes of spurious results	Heparin, levodopa, methyldopa, tolbutamide, p-aminosalicylic acid, erythromycin, diabetic ketoacidosis	Falsely elevated
Additional info	N/A	

Albumin

PARAMETER	DESCRIPTION	COMMENTS
Common reference range		
Adults	3.8–5 g/dL	
<1 yr old		
<2.5 kg	2.0–3.6 g/dL	
>2.5 kg	2.6–3.6 g/dL	
1–3 yr old	3.4–4.2 g/dL	
4–6 yr old	3.5–5.2 g/dL	
7–19 yr old	3.7–5.6 g/dL	
Critical value	<2.5 g/dL in adults	
Inherent activity	Yes	Increases oncotic pressure of plasma; carrier protein
Location		
Production	Liver	
Storage	Serum	
Secretion/ excretion	Broken down in liver	Half-life about 20 days
Causes of abnormal levels		
High	Anabolic steroids	
	Dehydration	
Low	Decreased hepatic synthesis, malnutrition or malabsorption	Seen in liver disease
	Protein losses	Substrate deficiency
	Pregnancy or chronic illness	Via kidney in nephrotic syndrome or via gut in protein-losing enteropathy
Signs and symptoms		
High level	N/A	
Low level	Edema, pulmonary edema, ascites	
After event, time until…		
Initial elevation	Days	
Peak values	Weeks	
Normalization	Days	
Causes of spurious results	Ampicillin, heparin, penicillin	Ampicillin and heparin may cause falsely elevated levels; penicillin may cause falsely lowered levels
Additional info	N/A	

Alkaline Phosphatase (ALP)

PARAMETER	DESCRIPTION	COMMENTS
Common reference range		
Adults	Varies with assay	Conditions that elevate ALP are found below
Pediatrics	Can be twofold to threefold higher than in adults	
Critical value	N/A	
Inherent activity	Yes	Intracellular activity only
Location		
Production	Intracellular enzyme	
Storage	Liver, placenta, bone, small intestine, leukocytes	These tissues are rich in ALP
Secretion/ excretion	None	
Causes of abnormal levels		
High	Cholestasis	Hepatic; associated with elevation of GGTP
	Bone	Paget's disease, bone tumors, rickets, osteomalacia, healing fracture
	Pregnancy	Placental ALP
	Childhood	Bone formation
Low	Vitamin D intoxication	
	Scurvy, hypothyroidism	
Signs and symptoms		
High level	N/A	
Low level	N/A	
After event, time until...		
Initial elevation	Hours	
Peak values	Days	
Normalization	Days	
Causes of spurious results	Blood drawn after fatty meal and prolonged serum storage	
Additional info	N/A	

Alpha Fetoprotein (AFp)

PARAMETER	DESCRIPTION	COMMENTS
Common reference range	<20 ng/mL	Pediatric range unknown
Critical value	N/A	
Inherent activity	Protein made normally during fetal and neonatal stages	Levels should decline after birth
Location	Liver and yolk cells	Detected in patient serum
Causes of abnormal levels		
High	Cancer (mainly liver and testicular); can be elevated in other cancers such as pancreatic, gastric, lung, and colon cancers as well as pregnancy, hepatitis, and cirrhosis	
Low	N/A	
Signs and symptoms		
High level	N/A	
Low level	N/A	
After event, time until…		
Normalization of levels	7 days	Event: surgical resection
		Elevated levels beyond 7 days suggests residual disease
Causes of spurious results	N/A	
Additional info	In the United States, used primarily to aid diagnosis of hepatocellular carcinoma	May be used to screen for liver cancer in parts of the world at increased risk for this malignancy

Aminoglycosides

PARAMETER	DESCRIPTION	COMMENTS
Common reference range	**Amikacin**	If dosing interval adjusted to 2–3 times half-life, steady state is reached after 3rd or 4th dose
	Traditional: peak 20–30 mg/L; trough 1–8 mg/L	
	Extended interval: trough undetectable	Peaks recommended within 30 min after end of infusion; troughs within 30 min before start of infusion
	Gentamicin/tobramycin	
	Traditional: peak 6–10 mg/L; trough 0.5–2 mg/L	
	Extended interval: trough undetectable	
Critical values	**Amikacin**	Peak levels associated with ototoxicity
	Peaks >35–40 mg/L for 7–10 days	
	Troughs >10 mg/L for sustained periods	Trough levels associated with nephrotoxicity
	Gentamicin/tobramycin	
	Peaks >12–14 mg/L for 7–10 days	
	Troughs >2–3 mg/L for sustained periods	
Inherent activity	Inhibits bacterial protein synthesis	
Location	N/A	
Causes of abnormal levels		
High	Renal impairment	
Low	Burns	
Signs and symptoms		
High level	High troughs: nephrotoxicity (acute tubular necrosis)	
	High peaks: ototoxicity	
Low level	N/A	
After event, time until...		
Normalization	Steady state varies with renal function	
Causes of spurious results	If patient is receiving beta-lactams and there is a delay to test the sample, a falsely low level may result	
	Tobra: doxycycline, cefoxitin, levodopa, rifampin	
Additional info	Efficacy related to peak concentration	
	Postantibiotic effects	

Ammonia

PARAMETER	DESCRIPTION	COMMENTS
Common reference range		
Adults and pediatrics	30–70 mcg/dL	Varies with assay
Newborn	90–150 mcg/dL	
Critical value	Generally 1.5 x ULN	
Inherent activity	Unknown	Progressive deterioration in neurologic function
Location		
Production	Gut (by bacteria)	
Storage	None	
Secretion/ excretion	Liver metabolizes to urea	Urea cycle; diminished in cirrhosis
Causes of abnormal levels		
High	Liver failure, Reye's syndrome, metabolic abnormalities	
Low	N/A	
Signs and symptoms		
High level	Hepatic encephalopathy	
Low level	N/A	
After event, time until…		
Initial elevation	Hours	
Peak values	No peak; rises progressively	
Normalization	Days	
Causes of spurious results	N/A	
Additional info	N/A	

Amphetamines and Methamphetamines (Urine Drug Screen)

PARAMETER	DESCRIPTION	COMMENTS
Common reference range	Negative	
Critical value	Positive	
Inherent activity	Yes	CNS stimulation
Location		
Production	N/A	
Storage	N/A	
Secretion/ excretion	N/A	
Causes of abnormal levels		
High	Ephedrine, pseudoephedrine, selegiline, chlorpromazine, trazodone, bupropion, desipramine, amantadine, ranitidine, phenylpropanolamine, methylenedioxymethamphetamine (MDMA), labetalol, phentermine, amphetamine/dextroamphetamine products	
Low	N/A	
Signs and symptoms		
High level	Hypertension, tachycardia, stroke, arrhythmias, cardiovascular collapse, rhabdomyolysis, hyperthermia, euphoria, irritability, insomnia, tremors, seizures, paranoia and aggressiveness	Symptoms related to overdose
Low level	N/A	
After event, time until…		
Negative result from sporadic use	2–5 days	Clearance is faster in acidic urine
Negative result from chronic use	Up to 2 wk	Methylphenidate typically will not be detected
Causes of spurious results	Mefenamic acid	May cause false-negative result
	Dietary supplements containing ephedra, phenylephrine, desoxyephedrine	May cause false-positive result
Additional info	N/A	

Amylase

PARAMETER	DESCRIPTION	COMMENTS
Common reference range	60–180 units/L	
Critical value	Unknown	May increase to 25 times upper limit of normal in acute pancreatitis
Inherent activity	Yes	Breaks starch into individual glucose molecules
Location		
Production	Pancreas/salivary glands	
Storage	Lungs, liver, fallopian tubes, ovaries, testes, small intestine, skeletal muscle, adipose tissue, thyroid, tonsils	
Secretion/ excretion	Kidney (25% of clearance)	Remaining mechanism of clearance not understood
Causes of abnormal levels		
High	Azathioprine, cimetidine, didanosine, estrogens, methyldopa, steroids, thiazides, HMG-COA reductase inhibitors	Didanosine routinely monitored
	Pancreatitis, hepatobiliary injury, perforated peptic ulcer, intestinal obstruction, ovarian or fallopian cysts, pregnancy, renal failure, diabetic ketoacidosis	
Low	N/A	
Signs and symptoms		
High level	Related to underlying cause	
Low level	N/A	
After event, time until…		
Initial elevation	2–6 hr	Event: acute pancreatitis
Peak values	12–30 hr	
Normalization	3–5 days	Assuming cause has been adequately treated
Causes of spurious results	Hypertriglyceridemia	May cause falsely low levels (but can also cause pancreatitis)
Additional info	N/A	

Anion Gap

PARAMETER	DESCRIPTION	COMMENTS
Common reference range	3–16 mEq/L	Institution dependent (12 mEq/L commonly cited as ULN due to improvements in electrolyte measurement)
Critical values	N/A	
Inherent activity	N/A	A calculation to estimate unmeasured anions; presence of anion gap suggests acidosis
Location	N/A	
Causes of abnormal levels		
High	Methanol, uremia, diabetic ketoacids, propylene glycol/paraldehyde, isoniazid, lactic acid, ethanol/ethylene glycol, salicylates	Calculated when evaluating causes of acidosis/intoxication
Low	Metabolic acidosis caused by production of HCl or loss of bicarbonate (e.g., carbonic anhydrase inhibitors, amphotericin B, lead, ammonium chloride, topiramate, RTA, diarrhea) commonly have low/normal anion gaps	
	Hypoalbuminemia, hyperlipidemia, lithium intoxication, multiple myeloma	
Signs and symptoms		
High level	Increased or decreased cardiac output, hyperkalemia, altered mental status, coma	
Low level	Dependent on underlying cause	
After event, time until…	N/A	
Causes of spurious results	Hypoalbuminemia, hyperlipidemia, multiple myeloma might mask AG acidosis	
Additional info	$AG = Na - (Cl + HCO_3)$	
	Urinary $AG = Na + K - Cl$ (all measured in urine)	
	If a positive value results from urinary AG calculation in a patient with nongap acidosis, suggests renal cause (if negative, bowel)	

Antifactor Xa Activity

PARAMETER	DESCRIPTION	COMMENTS
Common reference range		
Adults	0.5–1.1 units/mL	For twice daily therapeutic dosing of LMWH
	1–2 units/mL	For once daily therapeutic dosing of LMWH
		Values may vary depending on LMWH preparation used
Inherent activity	No	Measures ability of plasma sample to form a complex with factor Xa
Location		
Production	Coagulation factors produced in liver	
Storage	Not stored	
Secretion/ excretion	None	
Causes of abnormal levels		
High	Over dosage of LMWH, poor renal function	Used to monitor LMWH activity in underweight, obese, renal impairment
Low	Labs drawn prior to 4 hr after dose is administered, under dosing of LMWH	
Signs and symptoms		
High level	Increased risk of bleeding and bruising	
Low level	Potential thrombosis	
After event, time until…		
Initial elevation	0–4 hr	
Peak values	4 hr	
Normalization	Hours to days	
Causes of spurious results	Improper timing of collection	Peak level should be drawn 4 hr after dose is administered
Additional info	N/A	

Antinuclear Antibodies (ANA)

PARAMETER	DESCRIPTION	COMMENTS
Common reference range	Negative	Titer <1:40
Critical value	Titer: >1:320	Varies among laboratories
Inherent activity	Yes	Heterogeneous group of autoantibodies directed against nucleic acids and nucleoproteins within the nucleus and cytoplasm
Location		
Production	N/A	
Storage	Serum	
Secretion/excretion	N/A	
Causes of abnormal levels		
High	Idiopathic SLE, drug induced lupus, mixed connective-tissue disease	Rheumatic diseases
	Hashimoto's thyroiditis, idiopathic pulmonary fibrosis, primary pulmonary hypertension, idiopathic thrombocytopenic purpura, hemolytic anemia	Immunologic-mediated nonrheumatic diseases
	Bacterial, parasitic or viral infections, neoplasm	Nonimmunologic-mediated nonrheumatic diseases
Low	N/A	
Signs and symptoms		
High level	Related to underlying cause	
Low level	N/A	
After event, time until…		
Initial elevation	N/A	
Peak values	N/A	
Normalization	N/A	
Causes of spurious results	N/A	
Additional info	Low specificity makes ANAs testing unsuitable for use as a screening tool for rheumatic or nonrheumatic diseases in asymptomatic individuals	ANA is used as part of the diagnostic workup for symptomatic patients with suspected SLE

Antiphospholipid Antibodies

PARAMETER	DESCRIPTION	COMMENTS
Common reference range	Lupus anticoagulant: negative	
	Anticardiolipin antibody: ≤40	
	β_2 Glycoprotein I: ≤99th percentile	
Critical values	Lupus anticoagulant: positive	
	Anticardiolipin antibody: >40	
	β_2 Glycoprotein I: >99th percentile	
Inherent activity	Cause vasculopathy, thrombocytopenia, and thrombosis	
Location	Blood	
Causes of abnormal levels		
High	Rheumatic disorders including SLE	
Low	N/A	
Signs and symptoms		
High level	Thrombosis (including VTE, CVA, MI, and fetal loss)	
Low level	N/A	
After event, time until...	N/A	
Causes of spurious results	UFH and direct thrombin inhibitors can cause false positives (assay dependent)	Warfarin will not cause interference
Additional info	N/A	

Antithrombin

PARAMETER	DESCRIPTION	COMMENTS
Common reference range	80% to 130% of mean population value	Lower range if <6 mo old
		Multiple assay modalities exist (range variable)
Critical values	<80%	
Inherent activity	Combines with heparin to bind and inactivate clotting factors	
Location	Blood	
Causes of abnormal levels		
High	N/A	
Low	Genetic, liver disease, preeclampsia	Not commonly monitored with medications
Signs and symptoms		
High level	N/A	
Low level	VTE	
After event, time until…	N/A	
Causes of spurious results	Warfarin may cause false elevation and heparin may cause falsely low values	
Additional info	Previously termed antithrombin III	Commonly a functional assay is performed prior to an antigen assay

aPTT (Activated Partial Thromboplastin Time)

PARAMETER	DESCRIPTION	COMMENTS
Common reference range	22–38 sec (when no anticoagulation is desired)	May vary by reagent/instrument used
		If on UFH for treatment of DVT or PE, aim for 1.5–2.5 times control aPTT
Critical value	>70–100 sec	
Inherent activity	N/A	Used to monitor UFH activity
Location		
Production	Coagulation factors produced in liver	
Causes of abnormal levels		
High	UFH, direct thrombin inhibitors, warfarin	UFH, argatroban, lepirudin commonly monitored with test
	Deficiency of factors II, V, VIII, IX, X, XI, XII, HMWK, prekallikrein, fibrinogen presence of lupus anticoagulant, liver dysfunction, vitamin K deficiency, DIC	
Low	Labs drawn less than 6 hr after start of heparin infusion	
Signs and symptoms		
High level	Increased risk of hemorrhage	Risk increases as aPTT increases
Low level	Thrombosis	
After event, time until…		
Initial elevation	6–12 hr	Event: UFH administration
Peak values	Hours to days	
Normalization	Hours to days	
Causes of spurious results	Improper laboratory collection	
Additional info	Also known as PTT, measures intrinsic coagulation cascade	

Aspartate Aminotransferase (AST)

PARAMETER	DESCRIPTION	COMMENTS
Common reference range		
Adults	8–42 International Units/L	Varies with assay
Newborns/Infants	20–65 International Units/L	Varies with assay
Critical value	>80 International Units/L	2 times upper limit of normal
Inherent activity	Yes	Intracellular enzymatic activity
Location		
Production	Intracellular enzyme	
Storage	Liver, cardiac muscle, kidneys, brain, pancreas, lungs	These tissues are rich in AST
Secretion/ excretion	N/A	
Causes of abnormal levels		
High	Isoniazid, HMG-COA reductase inhibitors, allopurinol, methotrexate, ketoconazole, valproic acid	Listed medications are routinely monitored
	Hepatitis, hemolysis, muscular diseases, MI, renal infarction, pulmonary infarction, necrotic tumors	Elevated in any disease with hepatocyte inflammation (liver cells)
		Elevated in any disease with damage to tissues rich in enzyme
Low	N/A	
Signs and symptoms		
High level	Varies with underlying disease	Reflects tissue or organ damage
Low level	N/A	
After event, time until...		
Initial elevation	2–6 hr	
Peak values	24–48 hr (without further cell damage)	With extensive liver or cellular damage, levels can go up to thousands
Normalization	24–48 hr	Assumes insult removed and no ongoing damage
Causes of spurious results	Heparin, levodopa, methyldopa, tolbutamide, p-aminosalicylic acid, erythromycin, diabetic ketoacidosis	Falsely elevated
	Metronidazole, trifluoperazine, vitamin B6 deficiency	Falsely lowered
Additional info	N/A	

Band Neutrophils

PARAMETER	DESCRIPTION	COMMENTS
Common reference range	3% to 5%	
Critical value	N/A	
Inherent activity	Yes	Immature form of neutrophils
Location		
Production	Bone marrow	
Storage	Bone marrow, vascular endothelium	
Secretion/excretion	N/A	
Causes of abnormal levels		
High	Epinephrine, lithium, G-CSF, GM-CSF	G-CSF and GM-CSF commonly monitored
	Acute/chronic bacterial infection, trauma, MI, leukemia	
Low	Antineoplastic cytotoxic agents, captopril, cephalosporins, chloramphenicol, ganciclovir, methimazole, penicillins, phenothiazines, procainamide, ticlopidine, tricyclic antidepressants, vancomycin	Antineoplastic/cytotoxic agents, chloramphenicol, ganciclovir, methimazole, ticlopidine commonly monitored
	Radiation exposure, vitamin B12 or folate deficiency, salmonellosis, pertussis, overwhelming bacterial infection	
Signs and symptoms		
High level	Related to underlying cause	
Low level	Related to underlying cause	
After event, time until...		
Initial elevation	N/A	
Peak values	N/A	
Normalization	N/A	
Causes of spurious results	N/A	
Additional info	N/A	

Barbiturates (Urine Drug Screen)

PARAMETER	DESCRIPTION	COMMENTS
Common reference range	Negative	
Critical value	Positive	
Inherent activity	Yes	Sedation, muscle relaxation
Location		
Production	N/A	
Storage	N/A	
Secretion/excretion	N/A	
Causes of abnormal levels		
High	Primidone, phenobarbital	
Low	N/A	
Signs and symptoms		
High level	Coma, ataxia, nystagmus, depressed reflexes, hypotension, respiratory depression	Symptoms related to overdose
Low level	N/A	
After event, time until…		
Negative result from sporadic use	1–7 days	Depends on drug and duration of use
Negative result from chronic use	1–3 wk	Phenobarbital may be detected up to 4 wk after stopping use
Causes of spurious results	N/A	
Additional info	N/A	

Basophils

PARAMETER	DESCRIPTION	COMMENTS
Common reference range	0% to 1%	
Critical value	>300 cells/µL	
Inherent activity	Yes	Release histamine during allergic response
Location		
Production	Bone marrow	
Storage	Serum	
Secretion/ excretion	N/A	
Causes of abnormal levels		
High	Hypersensitivity reactions	Immediate or delayed
	Chronic inflammation	
	Leukemia	
Low	N/A	
Signs and symptoms		
High level	Related to underlying cause	
Low level	N/A	
After event, time until...		
Initial elevation	N/A	
Peak values	N/A	
Normalization	N/A	
Causes of spurious results	N/A	
Additional info	N/A	

BCR-ABL Fusion Gene

PARAMETER	DESCRIPTION	COMMENTS
Common reference range	N/A	This is an abnormal fusion gene that results from a genetic translocation producing a fusion mRNA normally not present in any significant amount unless a malignancy is present
Critical value	N/A	
Inherent activity	Causes abnormal growth of cells	Translocation results in an abnormal fusion protein with increased tyrosine kinase activity continually signaling cells to grow
Location	Derivative chromosome 22 resulting from t(9;22) translocation	Called the Philadelphia chromosome
Causes of abnormal levels		
High	Leukemias (CML, ALL, rarely AML)	
	mRNA levels can be determined quantitatively	
Low	Imatinib, dasatinib, nilotinib	Levels of BCR-ABL mRNA should decrease with these therapies; failure to do so indicates treatment failure
Signs and symptoms		
High level	N/A	
Low level	N/A	
After event, time until…	N/A	
Causes of spurious results	N/A	
Additional info	Rising levels of BCR-ABL mRNA correlate with increasing disease activity whereas falling levels are consistent with response to therapy	

Benzodiazepines (Urine Drug Screen)

PARAMETER	DESCRIPTION	COMMENTS
Common reference range	Negative	
Critical value	Positive	
Inherent activity	Yes	Drowsiness, ataxia, sedation
Location		
Production	N/A	
Storage	N/A	
Secretion/ excretion	N/A	
Causes of abnormal levels		
High	Ingestion or injection of benzodiazepines	
Low	Flunitrazepam (rohypnol)	May not be detected
Signs and symptoms		
High level	Tachycardia or bradycardia, coma, cardiovascular depression, respiratory depression	Symptoms related to overdose
Low level	N/A	
After event, time until…		
Negative result	Typically up to 2 wk	May take up to 6 wk with chronic use of some agents
Causes of spurious results	Not all benzodiazepines will be detected by all immunoassays	
Additional info	N/A	

Benzoylecgonine (Cocaine Metabolite) (Urine Drug Screen)

PARAMETER	DESCRIPTION	COMMENTS
Common reference range	Negative	
Critical value	Positive	
Inherent activity	Yes	CNS stimulation
Location		
Production	N/A	
Storage	N/A	
Secretion/ excretion	N/A	
Causes of abnormal levels		
High	Cocaine ingestion	
Low	N/A	
Signs and symptoms		
High level	Stroke, acute myocardial infarction, seizures, coma, respiratory depression, arrhythmias, dilated pupils, hyperthermia, tachycardia, and hypertension	
Low level	N/A	
After event, time until…		
Negative result from sporadic use	12–72 hr	
Negative result from chronic use	1–3 wk	
Causes of spurious results	Lidocaine, benzocaine, procaine	False positives are possible
	Topical anesthetics containing cocaine; coca leaf tea	
Additional info	Cross reactivity with cocaethylene (metabolic product of cocaine and ethanol abuse) varies with assay	

Beta-2-Microglobulin (B$_2$M)

PARAMETER	DESCRIPTION	COMMENTS
Common reference range	<2.5 mcg/mL	Pediatric range unknown
		Levels should decline after birth
Critical value	N/A	
Inherent activity	Unknown	
Location	Protein found on surface of lymphocytes and other MHC I molecules	Present in small amounts in the urine and blood
Causes of abnormal levels		
High	Multiple myeloma, lymphoma, and in renal failure	
Low	N/A	
Signs and symptoms		
High level	May see signs of renal failure or associated cancers	Renally excreted so elevated levels may indicate renal failure
Low level	N/A	
After event, time until…	N/A	
Causes of spurious results	N/A	
Additional info	Plays important role in staging and prognosis of multiple myeloma	

Bicarbonate (HCO₃)/Total CO₂ (Venous)

PARAMETER	DESCRIPTION	COMMENTS
Common reference range		
Adults	HCO_3: 24–30 mEq/L	TCO_2 ranges may be 0–2 mEq/L higher
Preterm infants	HCO_3: 16–20 mEq/L	
Full-term infants	HCO_3: 19–21 mEq/L	
Infants/children (2 yr old)	HCO_3: 18–28 mEq/L	
Critical values	<8 mEq/L	
Inherent activity	Major extracellular anion, part of buffer system	
Location	Reflects amount of HCO_3 in venous blood	
Causes of abnormal levels		
High	Loop diuretics, steroids, excess bicarbonate therapy	HCO_3 occasionally monitored with chronic loop diuretic, $NaHCO_3$, and topiramate administration and daily with frequent hospital titration
	Metabolic alkalosis, compensation for respiratory alkalosis	
Low	Salicylate overdose, carbonic anhydrase inhibitors, topiramate	
	Metabolic acidosis, compensation for respiratory acidosis	
Signs and symptoms		
High level	Arteriolar constriction, hypokalemia, seizures, lethargy, stupor	
Low level	Decreased cardiac output, hyperkalemia, altered mental status, coma	
After event, time until…		
Normalization	Respiratory compensation: minutes to hours	
Causes of spurious results	N/A	
Additional info	Technically, there are methods to directly measure bicarbonate, but commonly the bicarbonate will be converted to CO_2 and measured as TCO_2	Bicarbonate represents ~95% of the CO_2 in the TCO_2 sample; often, TCO_2 is referred to as bicarbonate in clinical situations

Blood Urea Nitrogen (BUN)

PARAMETER	DESCRIPTION	COMMENTS
Common reference range	8–20 mg/dL	
Critical value	>100 mg/dL	Associated with higher risk of uremic syndrome
Inherent activity	N/A	
Location		
Production	Liver	Urea production
Storage	Serum	
Secretion/ excretion	Kidney	
Causes of abnormal levels		
High	Corticosteroids, tetracycline	Listed medications not commonly monitored
	High protein diet (including amino acid infusions)	
	Upper GI bleed	
	Decreased renal perfusion	Dehydration, blood loss, shock, severe heart failure
	Acute kidney failure	Severe hypertension, glomerulonephritis, tubular necrosis
	Chronic kidney dysfunction	Pyelonephritis, diabetes, amyloidosis, polycystic kidney disease
	Obstruction	Ureter, bladder or urethra
Low	Malnutrition, profound liver disease	Unable to synthesize urea
Signs and symptoms		
High level	Related to underlying disorder	
Low level	Related to underlying disorder	
After event, time until…		
Initial elevation	N/A	
Peak values	N/A	
Normalization	N/A	
Causes of spurious results	N/A	
Additional info	BUN:SCr ratio greater than 20:1 suggest prerenal cause of kidney injury	

B-Type Natriuretic Peptide (BNP) & NT-proBNP

PARAMETER	DESCRIPTION	COMMENTS
Common reference range	BNP: <100 pg/mL NT-proBNP: males <61 pg/mL females 12–151 pg/mL	
Critical value	BNP: >100 pg/mL NT-proBNP: >125 pg/mL if age <75 >450 pg/mL if age >75	Affected by age, gender, renal function, and obesity
Inherent activity	BNP: yes NT-proBNP: no	Diuretic, natriuretic, and vascular smooth muscle-relaxing effects
Location		
Production/storage	Ventricular myocyte	Released in response to increased ventricular wall tension
Secretion/excretion	BNP: enzymatic degradation via endopeptidase and endocytosis NT-proBNP: renal elimination	
Causes of abnormal levels		
High	Heart failure, PE, pulmonary diseases	
Low	N/A	
Signs and symptoms		
High level	Shortness of breath, edema	
Low level	N/A	
After event, time until…	N/A	
Causes of spurious results	Renal impairment, obesity	Levels of NT-proBNP might be falsely high in patients with renal impairment Levels of NT-proBNP may be falsely low in obese patients
Additional info	proBNP is cleaved to form active BNP and inactive NT-proBNP	

C3 and C4

PARAMETER	DESCRIPTION	COMMENTS
Common reference range	C3: 72–156 mg/dL	
	C4: 20–50 mg/dL	
Critical value	N/A	
Inherent activity	Yes	Primary role is the destruction of microbes
Location		
Production	Liver	
Storage	Serum	
Secretion/ excretion	N/A	
Causes of abnormal levels		
High	Cimetidine, cyclophosphamide	Listed medications are not commonly monitored
	Rheumatoid arthritis, malignancy	
Low	Systemic lupus erythematosus, systemic vasculitis, viral infections, parasitic infections	
Signs and symptoms		
High level	Related to underlying cause	
Low level	Related to underlying cause	
After event, time until…		
Initial elevation	N/A	
Peak values	N/A	
Normalization	N/A	
Causes of spurious results	N/A	
Additional info	Results of C3 and C4 are helpful in following patients who present with low levels and then undergo treatment	

CA 125 (Cancer Antigen 125)

PARAMETER	DESCRIPTION	COMMENTS
Common reference range	<35 units/mL	Pediatric range unknown
Critical value	Levels >65 units/mL consistent with malignancy (but not diagnostic)	Levels <10 units/mL associated with favorable prognosis
Inherent activity	Unknown	
Location	Protein found on cells of the pelvic peritoneum	Detected in serum of patients
Causes of abnormal levels		
High	Cancer (mainly ovarian, cervical, and fallopian tube cancers), endometriosis, ovarian cysts, liver disease, pregnancy, menstruation	
Low	Oral contraceptives	Oral contraceptives not commonly monitored with test
	Luteal phase of cycle, menopausal women	
Signs and symptoms		
High level	N/A	
Low level	N/A	
After event, time until…	N/A	
Causes of spurious results	N/A	
Additional info	Used to detect recurrence/residual disease of ovarian cancer after resection	

CA 15-3 (Cancer Antigen 15-3)

PARAMETER	DESCRIPTION	COMMENTS
Common reference range	<25 units/mL	Pediatric range unknown
Critical value	N/A	
Inherent activity	Unknown	
Location	Serum	
Storage	Unknown	
Secretion/ excretion	Secreted from breast tissue	Antibody detects circulating mucin antigen secreted
Causes of abnormal levels		
High	Breast cancer, may be elevated in other cancers of lung, colon, ovary and pancreas origin and benign breast disorders	
Low	N/A	
Signs and symptoms		
High level	N/A	
Low level	N/A	
After event, time until…	N/A	
Causes of spurious results	N/A	
Additional info	Poor prognostic factor for patients with early stage breast cancer	

CA 19-9 (Cancer Antigen 19-9)

PARAMETER	DESCRIPTION	COMMENTS
Common reference range	<37 units/mL	Pediatric range unknown
Critical value	N/A	
Inherent activity	Unknown	
Location	Pancreas, gastric cells, colon	Detected in serum
Causes of abnormal levels		
High	Pancreatic, gastric, and colon cancers; also in benign pancreatic disorders	
Low	N/A	
Signs and symptoms		
High level	N/A	
Low level	N/A	
After event, time until...	N/A	
Causes of spurious results	N/A	
Additional info	Recommended to evaluate treatment response and recurrence in patients with pancreatic cancer as well as distinguish pancreatic cancer from other pancreatic disease	Originally developed for colon cancer monitoring but no longer recommended

CA 27.29 (Cancer Antigen 27.29)

PARAMETER	DESCRIPTION	COMMENTS
Common reference range	<38 units/mL	Pediatric range unknown
Critical value	N/A	
Inherent activity	Unknown	
Location	Serum	
Storage	N/A	
Secretion/ excretion	Secreted from breast tissue	Antibody detects circulating mucin antigen secreted
Causes of abnormal levels		
High	Breast cancer, may be elevated in benign breast disorders	
Low	N/A	
Signs and symptoms		
High level	N/A	
Low level	N/A	
After event, time until…	N/A	
Causes of spurious results	N/A	
Additional info	May be useful for patients with metastatic breast cancer	
	Not useful as screening test for detection of recurrence after therapy for early stage breast cancer	

Calcium

PARAMETER	DESCRIPTION	COMMENTS
Common reference range		
Adults	8.5–10.8 mg/dL (2.1–2.7 mmol/L)	~½ bound to serum proteins; only ionized (free) calcium is active
	Ionized: 4.4–5.3 mg/dL	
Newborns (3–24 hr old)	9–10.6 mg/dL (2.3–2.65 mmol/L)	
	Ionized: 4.3–5.1 mg/dL	
Newborns (24–48 hr old)	7.0–12.0 mg/dL (1.75–3.0 mmol/L)	
	Ionized: 4.0-4.7 mg/dL	
Newborns (4–7 days old)	9.0–10.9 mg/dL (2.25–2.73 mmol/L)	
	Ionized: 4.5–4.92 mg/dL	
Children	8.8–10.8 mg/dL (2.2–2.7 mmol/L)	
	Ionized: 4.5–4.92 mg/dL	
Critical value	>14 or <7 mg/dL (>3.5 or <1.8 mmol/L)	Also depends on serum albumin and pH values
Inherent activity	Yes	Preservation of cellular membranes, propagation of neuromuscular activity, regulation of endocrine functions, blood coagulation, bone metabolism
Location		
Storage	99.5% in bone and teeth	Very closely regulated
Secretion/ excretion	Filtration by kidneys	Small amounts excreted into GI tract from saliva, bile, and pancreatic/intestinal secretions
Causes of abnormal levels		
High	Thiazide diuretics, lithium, vitamin D, calcium supplements	Listed drugs are commonly monitored
	Malignancy, hyperparathyroidism	
Low	Loop diuretics, calcitonin, bisphosphonates	Listed drugs are commonly monitored
	Vitamin D deficiency, CKD, hypoparathyroidism, hyperphosphatemia, pancreatitis	

(continued)

Calcium (Cont.)

Signs and symptoms		
High level	GI complaints, neurologic and cardiovascular sx, ventricular arrhythmias, renal dysfunction, vascular calcification	More severe with acute onset
Low level	Neuromuscular (fatigue, depression, memory loss, hallucinations, seizures, tetany), QT prolongation	More severe with acute onset
After event, time until…		
Initial elevation	Variable	Faster change is more dangerous
Peak values	Variable	
Normalization	Days, if renal function is normal	Faster with appropriate treatment
Causes of spurious results	Hypoalbuminemia	Ionized calcium concentration usually unaffected
Additional info	Corrected Ca = measured Ca + [0.8*(4-albumin)]	Measurement of ionized calcium negates the need to correct for hypoalbuminemia

Carbamazepine

PARAMETER	DESCRIPTION	COMMENTS
Common reference range	4–12 mg/L	Trough level recommended
	4–8 mg/L if concomitant primidone, phenobarbital, valproic acid or phenytoin	
Critical values	>15 mg/L associated with ADRs	
	>50 mg/L associated with serious ADRs	
Inherent activity	Anticonvulsant and mood-stabilizing actions	
Location	N/A	
Causes of abnormal levels		
High	Carbamazepine	Levels not commonly monitored
	3A4 inhibitors	
Low	Diseases causing decreased protein binding may cause falsely low levels	
	3A4 inducers	
Signs and symptoms		
High level	N/V, unsteadiness, blurred vision, drowsiness, headache	
Low level	N/A	
After event, time until…		
Normalization	2–3 wk until steady-state	
Causes of spurious results	Doxycycline, levodopa, methyldopa, and metronidazole can cause false positives	
Additional info	Patients taking primidone, phenobarbital, valproic acid, or phenytoin may accumulate active metabolite	Autoinduction causes variable half-life

Carcinoembryonic Antigen (CEA)

PARAMETER	DESCRIPTION	COMMENTS
Common reference range	<2.5 ng/mL	<5.0 ng/mL for smokers Pediatric normal range unknown
Critical value	N/A	
Inherent activity	Unknown	
Location	Intestine, pancreas, liver	Normally found during fetal development only; detected in serum of patients
Causes of abnormal levels		
High	Cancer (mainly colon), smoking, hepatitis, pancreatitis, peptic ulcer disease, hypothyroidism, ulcerative colitis, Crohn's disease	Usually <10 ng/mL in nonmalignant conditions
Low	N/A	
Signs and symptoms		
High level	N/A	
Low level	N/A	
After event, time until…	N/A	
Causes of spurious results	N/A	
Additional info	Limited sensitivity and specificity Used to evaluate response to some chemotherapy	

CD4⁺ T Lymphocyte Count

PARAMETER	DESCRIPTION	COMMENTS
Common reference range	800–1100 cells/mm³ 40% of total lymphocytes	
Critical value	<200 cells/mm³ <14% of total lymphocytes	
Inherent activity	Yes	Helper inducer T cells
Location		
Production	Bone marrow	
Storage	Thymus Serum	
Secretion/excretion	N/A	
Causes of abnormal levels		
High	N/A	
Low	Severe immunosuppression due to HIV infection	Patient is at high risk of developing opportunistic infections
Signs and symptoms		
High level	N/A	
Low level	Related to progression of HIV	
After event, time until…		
Initial elevation	N/A	
Peak values	N/A	
Normalization	N/A	
Causes of spurious results	N/A	
Additional info	Provides an estimate of the patient's immune status	
	Essential component of the management of patients with HIV-1 infection	
	Used in conjunction with the HIV-RNA level to provide essential information regarding the patients' immunologic and virologic status, risk of disease progression to AIDS, and whether to initiate or change antiretroviral therapy	

Chloride

PARAMETER	DESCRIPTION	COMMENTS
Common reference range	96–106 mEq/L (96–106 mmol/L)	
Critical value	N/A	Depends on underlying disorder
Inherent activity	Yes	Primary anion in ECF and gastric fluid, cardiac function, acid base balance
Location		
Storage	ECF	Most abundant extracellular anion
Secretion/ excretion	Passively follows sodium and water	Influenced by acid-base balance
Causes of abnormal levels		
High	Dehydration, acidemia, diarrhea	
Low	Diuretics	
	Nasogastric suction, vomiting, serum dilution, alkalemia	
Signs and symptoms		
High level	Associated with underlying disorder	
Low level	Associated with underlying disorder	
After event, time until…		
Initial elevation	Variable	
Peak values	Variable	
Normalization	Days, if renal function is normal	
Causes of spurious results	Bromides and iodides (falsely elevated)	
Additional info	N/A	

Chromium

PARAMETER	DESCRIPTION	COMMENTS
Common reference range		
Adults	1–5 mcg/L (18–92 nmol/L)	Analysis of chromium in biological fluids and tissues is difficult
Pediatrics	Unknown	Analysis of chromium in biological fluids and tissues is difficult
Critical value	N/A	
Inherent activity	Yes	Cofactor for insulin and metabolism of glucose, cholesterol, and triglycerides
Location		
Storage	Hair, kidneys, bone, liver, spleen, lungs, testes, large intestines	Chromium circulates as free Cr^{3+}, bound to transferrin and other proteins, and as organic complex
Secretion/excretion	Excretion in urine	Circulating insulin may affect excretion
Causes of abnormal levels		
High	Chromium supplement, possibly during chronic TPN	Serum chromium concentration not routinely monitored
Low	Decreased intake	
Signs and symptoms		
High level	N/A	
Low level	Glucose intolerance; hyperinsulinemia; hypercholesterolemia; possibly, risk of cardiovascular disease	Mainly due to its role as insulin cofactor
After event, time until…	N/A	
Causes of spurious results	N/A	
Additional info	N/A	

CK-MB Isoenzyme Subforms (CK-MB$_1$ and CK-MB$_2$)

PARAMETER	DESCRIPTION	COMMENTS
Common reference range	0.5–1 units/L for each subform	CK-MB$_2$ and CK-MB$_1$ in equilibrium
Critical value	CK-MB$_2$: 1 units/L CK-MB$_2$: CK-MB$_1$ ratio: 1.5	CK-MB$_2$ and ratio increase soon after AMI until new equilibrium reached
Inherent activity	CK-MB$_1$: unknown CK-MB$_2$: yes	CKMB$_2$ catalyzes final step of glycolysis
Location		
Production	Heart and skeletal muscle	
Storage	Not stored	
Secretion/excretion	Excreted via glomerular filtration	
Causes of abnormal levels		
High	MI, pericarditis, myositis, vigorous exercise, surgery, hyper/hypothermia, hypothyroidism, renal failure, subarachnoid hemorrhage, muscular dystrophy	
Low	N/A	No lower limit for normal
Signs and symptoms		
High level	Chest pain, N/V, diaphoresis	Decreased or increased HR and BP, anxiety, and confusion depending on MI size, location, and duration
Low level	N/A	Does not cause signs and symptoms
After event, time until…		
Initial elevation	2–4 hr	Event: MI Sooner with non-Q-wave MI as early use of thrombolytic agent
Peak values	6–8 hr	Sooner with non-Q-wave MI as early use of thrombolytic agent
Normalization	10–14 days	Sooner with non-Q-wave MI as early use of thrombolytic agent
Causes of spurious results	N/A	
Additional info	CK-MB$_2$ found in myocardial cells CK-MB$_1$ formed from CK-MB$_2$ in plasma after in vivo loss of terminal lysine Assays not widely available	

CK-MB Isoenzymes

PARAMETER	DESCRIPTION	COMMENTS
Common reference range	<12 International Units/L 0–5.9 ng/mL <3% to 6% of total CK	Assay dependent
Critical value	12 International Units/L >6% of total CK >5.9 ng/mL	Assay dependent
Inherent activity	Yes	Catalyzes transfer of high-energy phosphate groups
Location		
Production	Primarily cardiac muscle	Release from traumatized skeletal muscle can be incorrectly interpreted as cardiac in origin
Storage	Small amounts in skeletal muscle	
Secretion/excretion	Excreted via glomerular filtration	Eliminated at slightly faster rate than total CK
Causes of abnormal levels		
High	MI, pericarditis, myositis, vigorous exercise, surgery, hyper/hypothermia, hypothyroidism, renal failure, subarachnoid hemorrhage	
Low	N/A	No lower limit for normal
Signs and symptoms		
High level	MI: chest pain, N/V, diaphoresis	Abnormal HR and BP, anxiety, and confusion depending on MI size, location, and duration
Low level	N/A	Does not cause signs and symptoms
After event, time until…		
Initial elevation	3–12 hr	Event: MI Sooner with non-Q-wave MI or early use of thrombolytic agent
Peak values	12–20 hr	Sooner with non-Q-wave MI or early use of thrombolytic agent
Normalization	2–3 days	Sooner with non-Q-wave MI or early use of thrombolytic agent
Causes of spurious results	Isoenzyme variant, nonspecific fluorescence, spillover of CK-MM, doxycycline	Assay dependent
Additional into	N/A	

Complement Hemolytic 50%

PARAMETER	DESCRIPTION	COMMENTS
Common reference range	100–250 International Units/mL	
Critical value	<10 International Units/mL	
Inherent activity	None	
Location		
Production	N/A	
Storage	N/A	
Secretion/excretion	N/A	
Causes of abnormal levels		
High	N/A	
Low	SLE, anticardiolipin syndrome, Sjögren's syndrome, MCTD, vasculitis, mixed cryoglobulinemia, serum sickness, some glomerulonephritides including poststreptococcal nephritis	
Signs and symptoms		
High level	N/A	
Low level	Related to underlying cause	
After event, time until...		
Initial elevation	N/A	
Peak values	N/A	
Normalization	N/A	
Causes of spurious results	Improper specimen handling	False depressions
Additional info	Measures the ability of the patient's serum to lyse 50% of a standard suspension of sheep erythrocytes coated with rabbit antibody	
	All nine components of the classical pathway are required to produce a normal reaction	

Coombs' Test (Direct)

PARAMETER	DESCRIPTION	COMMENTS
Common reference range	Negative	
Critical values	Positive	
Inherent activity	N/A	Tests blood for antibodies directed at blood
Location	N/A	
Causes of abnormal levels		
High	Sulfonamides, nitrofurantoin, phenazopyridine, primaquine, dapsone in patients with G6PD	Not commonly monitored with listed medications unless hemolysis suspected
	Autoimmune hemolysis, lack of blood compatibility	
Low	N/A	
Signs and symptoms		
High level	Jaundice, discoloration of urine (brown), splenomegaly	
Low level	N/A	
After event, time until...	N/A	
Causes of spurious results	Drug-induced antibodies including isoniazid, sulfonamides, quinidine, methyldopa, cephalosporins	
Additional info	Used to assess autoimmune hemolysis and screen for blood transfusion compatibility	

Copper

PARAMETER	DESCRIPTION	COMMENTS
Common reference range		
Adults	65–155 mcg/dL (10–24.6 μmol/L)	
Pediatrics	20–70 mcg/dL (3.1–11 μmol/L)	0–6 mo
	90–190 mcg/dL (14.2–29.9 μmol/L)	6 yr
	80–160 mcg/dL (12.6–25.2 μmol/L)	12 yr
Critical value	N/A	
Inherent activity	Yes	Companion to iron enzyme cofactor, Hgb synthesis, collagen and elastin synthesis, metabolism of many neurotransmitters, energy generation, regulation of plasma lipid levels, cell protection against oxidative damage
Location		
Storage	⅓ in liver and brain; ⅓ in muscles; the rest in heart, spleen, kidneys, and blood (erythrocytes and neutrophils)	95% of circulating copper is protein bound as ceruloplasmin
Secretion/ excretion	Mainly by biliary excretion; only 0.5% to 3% of daily intake found in urine	
Causes of abnormal levels		
High	Copper supplements, possibly during chronic TPN	Serum copper concentrations not routinely monitored
	Deliberate ingestion of large amounts (>15 mg of elemental copper), Wilson's disease, uncommon in humans	
Low	Infants with chronic diarrhea, malabsorption syndromes, decreased intake over months, Menkes syndrome	
Signs and symptoms		
High level	N/V, intestinal cramps, diarrhea	Larger ingestions lead to shock, hepatic necrosis, intravascular hemolysis, renal impairment, coma, and death
Low level	Neutropenia, iron-deficiency anemia, abnormal glucose tolerance, arrhythmias, hypercholesterolemia, atherosclerosis, depressed immune function, defective connective tissue formation, demineralization of bones	Can affect any system or organ whose enzymes require copper for proper functioning
After event time to…	N/A	
Causes of spurious results	N/A	
Additional info	N/A	

Cortisol (Urine)

PARAMETER	DESCRIPTION	COMMENTS
Common reference range	20–90 mcg/dL	24-hr urine free collection
Critical value	>200 mcg/dL	
Inherent activity	Yes	Regulates fat, protein, and carbohydrate metabolism
Location		
Production	Adrenal gland	
Secretion/ excretion	Renal	
Causes of abnormal levels		
High	Corticosteroids can cross-react with some assays	
	Adrenocorticotropic hormone secreting tumor, adrenal tumors	
Low	Phenytoin, phenobarbital, rifampin, ketoconazole, corticosteroids	Levels not commonly monitored with listed medications
	Autoimmune, tuberculosis, acquired immunodeficiency syndrome (AIDS), fungal infections, amyloidosis	
Signs and symptoms		
High level	Facial plethora, fat accumulation, central obesity, hypertension, osteoporosis, depression, myopathies	
Low level	Weakness, weight loss, hypotension, postural dizziness, vertigo, gastrointestinal symptoms	
After event, time until...		
Initial elevation	N/A	
Peak values	N/A	
Normalization	N/A	
Causes of spurious results	N/A	
Additional info	N/A	

Cosyntropin Stimulation Test

PARAMETER	DESCRIPTION	COMMENTS
Common reference range	>18 mcg/dL	Serum cortisol level
Critical value	<9 mcg/dL	
Inherent activity	Yes	Stimulates cortisol production
Location		
Production/storage	N/A	
Secretion/excretion	N/A	
Causes of abnormal levels		
High	N/A	
Low	Phenytoin, phenobarbital, rifampin	Induce cortisol metabolism
	Ketoconazole	
	Corticosteroids	Inhibits cortisol production
	Autoimmune, tuberculosis, acquired immunodeficiency syndrome (AIDS), fungal infections, amyloidosis	HPA axis suppression
Signs and symptoms		
High level	N/A	
Low level	N/A	
After event, time until…		
Initial elevation	30–60 min	
Peak values	30–60 min	
Normalization	Hours	
Causes of spurious results	Acute illness	Elevated levels
Additional info	Cortisol levels measured at baseline and 30–60 min following administration of cosyntropin	

C-Peptide

PARAMETER	DESCRIPTION	COMMENTS
Common reference range	Fasting: 0.78–1.89 ng/mL	
	1 hr after glucose load: 5–12 ng/mL	
Critical value	N/A	
Inherent activity	Unknown	
Location		
Production	Pancreas	Proinsulin is synthesized and split into insulin and c-peptide
Storage	N/A	
Secretion/ excretion	Kidneys	
Causes of abnormal levels		
High	High levels of endogenous insulin production (may be caused by glucose intake or insulin resistance), insulinomas, impaired kidney function	
Low	Insufficient insulin production (e.g., Type I DM)	
Signs and symptoms		
High level	N/A	
Low level	N/A	
After event, time until…	N/A	
Causes of spurious results	N/A	
Additional info	N/A	

C-Reactive Protein (CRP)

PARAMETER	DESCRIPTION	COMMENTS
Common reference range	0–0.5 mg/dL	
Critical value	>1 mg/dL	Associated with inflammatory process
	>10 mg/dL	Associated with bacterial infection
Inherent activity	No specific function identified	
Location		
Production	N/A	
Storage	Serum	
Secretion/ excretion	N/A	
Causes of abnormal levels		
High	Inflammatory process, bacterial infection, atherosclerotic plaque, rheumatic disease	
Low	N/A	
Signs and symptoms		
High level	Related to underlying disease	
Low level	N/A	
After event, time until…		
Initial elevation	N/A	
Peak values	N/A	
Normalization	N/A	
Causes of spurious results	Lipemia, hemolysis	False-positive results
Additional info	Reflects immune system activity	

Creatine Kinase (CK)

PARAMETER	DESCRIPTION	COMMENTS
Common reference range		
Adults	Males: 40–200 International Units/L	Females lower due to smaller muscle mass
	Females: 35–150 International Units/L	
Pediatrics	>6 wk = adult value	
Critical value	150–200 International Units/L without signs and symptoms warrants further evaluation	At >70 International Units/L, some laboratories automatically test for CK-MB
Inherent activity	Yes	Catalyzes transfer of high-energy phosphate groups
Location		
Production	Skeletal and cardiac muscle and brain	
Storage	Not stored	
Secretion/ excretion	Excreted via glomerular filtration	Elimination may decrease in renal failure
Causes of abnormal levels		
High	Statins, amphotericin B, fibrates, niacin, ethanol, lithium, succinylcholine, barbiturates	
	IM injections	
	Skeletal muscle: myositis, trauma, seizures, vigorous exercise, rhabdomyolysis	
	Cardiac: myocarditis, pericarditis, MI	
	Other: hypothyroidism, renal failure, CVA, PE, severe hypokalemia	
Low	Abnormally low muscle mass	
	Cachexia and neuromuscular disease	

(continued)

Creatine Kinase (CK) (Cont.)

Signs and symptoms		
High level	MI: chest pain, N/V, diaphoresis, muscle cramps	Decreased or increased HR and BP, anxiety, and confusion, depending on MI size, location, and duration
Low level	Dependent on cause of abnormally low muscle mass	Does not cause signs and symptoms directly
After event, time until...		
Initial elevation	6–8 hr	Event: MI
		Sooner with non-Q-wave MI or early use of thrombolytic agent
Peak values	24 hr	Sooner with non-Q-wave MI or early use of thrombolytic agent
Normalization	3–4 days	Sooner with non-Q-wave MI or early use of thrombolytic agent
Causes of spurious results	N/A	
Additional info	Total CK measures composite of CK-MM, CK-MB, and CK-BB	

Cyclosporine

PARAMETER	DESCRIPTION	COMMENTS
Common reference range	100–400 mcg/L	Trough level recommended
	Up to 500 mcg/L if high risk for rejection (e.g., African Americans)	Some data to suggest 2-hr postdose levels are useful
		Range dependent on assay modality (whole blood reference range provided), indication, and time from transplant
Critical values	>400 mcg/L	
Inherent activity	Immunosuppressant	
Location	N/A	
Causes of abnormal levels		
High	Hypercholesterolemia and acute rejection can cause false elevation (higher proportion bound)	
	Drugs inhibiting 3A4	
Low	Hypocholesterolemia can cause falsely low levels (higher proportion unbound)	
	Drugs inducing 3A4	
Signs and symptoms		
High level	Nephrotoxicity, neurotoxicity, HTN, dyslipidemia, hirsutism, gingival hyperplasia	Levels should be monitored in everyone taking cyclosporine
Low level	N/A	
After event, time until…		
Normalization	Up to 5 days until steady state	
Causes of spurious results	Cholesterol levels	
Additional info	N/A	

D-Dimer

PARAMETER	DESCRIPTION	COMMENTS
Common reference range	<0.5 mcg/mL	
Critical values	N/A	
Inherent activity	No	Formed as degradation product of fibrin
Location	Produced at location of clot	
Causes of abnormal levels		
High	VTE, DIC, arterial thromboembolic disease, sepsis, CHF, malignancy, renal disease, pregnancy	
Low	N/A	
Signs and symptoms		
High level	Dependent on cause (no inherent symptoms)	
Low level	N/A	
After event, time until…	N/A	
Causes of spurious results	N/A	
Additional info	Sensitive, but not specific for VTE and DIC D-dimer is less sensitive than fibrin degradation products assay for DIC	Some studies evaluate D-dimer and duration of anticoagulation, but more studies needed

Delta-9-Tetrahydrocannabinol-9-Carbozylic Acid (THC) (Urine Drug Screen)

PARAMETER	DESCRIPTION	COMMENTS
Common reference range	Negative	
Critical value	Positive	
Inherent activity	Yes	
Location		
Production	N/A	
Storage	N/A	
Secretion/excretion	N/A	
Causes of abnormal levels		
High	Smoking or ingestion, dronabinol	
Low	N/A	
Signs and symptoms		
High level	Delirium, conjunctivitis, food craving, problems with memory and learning, distorted perception, difficulty problem solving, loss of coordination, sedation, tachycardia	
Low level	N/A	
After event, time until…		
Negative result from sporadic use	7–10 days	
Negative result from chronic use	6–8 wk up to 3 mo	May persist for longer period of time with heavy long-term use
Causes of spurious results	Ibuprofen, naproxen, efavirenz, hemp oil	False-positive result
Additional info	N/A	

Digoxin

PARAMETER	DESCRIPTION	COMMENTS
Common reference range	0.5–1 mcg/L heart failure	Draw at least 6 hr after dose to allow distribution
	1–2 mcg/L arrhythmias	
	1–2.6 mcg/L in neonates	
Critical values	>2.5 mcg/L	50% of patients have some digoxin toxicity above this level
Inherent activity	Inotropic and chronotropic effects on heart	
Location	N/A	
Causes of abnormal levels		
High	Renal impairment, elderly, medications that reduce clearance (amiodarone, verapamil, spironolactone, cyclosporine) or reduce metabolism (quinidine)	Levels commonly monitored for efficacy/toxicity
Low	Medications reducing absorption of digoxin (St John's wort, sulfasalazine, antacids)	
Signs and symptoms		
High level	Muscle weakness, N/V, constipation, confusion, HA, vertigo, change in color vision (yellow halos), AV block, bradycardia, ventricular tachycardia	
Low level	N/A	
After event, time until…		
Normalization	Up to 7 days until steady state	
Causes of spurious results	Toxicity greater when hypokalemic, hypomagnesemic, hypercalcemic, or in patients with structural heart disease	Ultrafiltration of a sample with digoxin-immune Fab fragments allows somewhat reliable level of unbound digoxin
	Hyperthyroidism reduces effect of digoxin	
	Levels drawn <10 days after digoxin-immune Fab fragment administration results in falsely high levels	
	Spironolactone may cause falsely low readings	
	Digoxin-like immunoreactive substance occurs naturally in some patients and causes falsely low levels	
Additional info	N/A	

Eosinophils

PARAMETER	DESCRIPTION	COMMENTS
Common reference range	0% to 4%	
Critical value	>350 cells/μL	
	<50 cells/μL	
Inherent activity	Yes	Phagocytize, kill, and digest bacteria and yeast
Location		
Production	Bone marrow	
Storage	Intestinal mucosa, lungs	
Secretion/excretion	N/A	
Causes of abnormal levels		
High	ACE-I, drug allergy	Monitored if symptoms suggest allergic response
	Allergic disorders, asthma, leukemia, parasitic infections, interstitial nephritis	
Low	Acute infection	
Signs and symptoms		
High level	Related to underlying cause	
Low level	Related to underlying cause	
After event, time until…		
Initial elevation	N/A	
Peak values	N/A	
Normalization	N/A	
Causes of spurious results	N/A	
Additional info	N/A	

Erythrocyte Sedimentation Rate (ESR)

PARAMETER	DESCRIPTION	COMMENTS
Common reference range		
Adults (Westergren method)		
Males		
<50 years old	<15 mm/hr	
>50 years old	<20 mm/hr	
Females		
<50 years old	<20 mm/hr	
>50 years old	<30 mm/hr	
Children		
Newborn	0–2 mm/hr	
Neonatal-puberty	3–13 mm/hr	
Critical value	>50 mm/hr	
Inherent activity	N/A	
Location		
Production	N/A	
Storage	N/A	
Secretion/excretion	N/A	
Causes of abnormal levels		
High	Obesity, increased age, rheumatic disease	Polymyalgia rheumatic, temporal arteritis
	Inflammatory process, infectious process, pregnancy	
Low	N/A	
Signs and symptoms		
High level	Related to underlying cause	
Low level	N/A	
After event, time until...		
Initial elevation	N/A	
Peak values	N/A	
Normalization	Days to weeks	Assuming underlying cause has been treated appropriately
Causes of spurious results	N/A	
Additional info	Measures the rate at which erythrocytes suspended in plasma fall when placed in a vertical tube	

Estradiol

PARAMETER	DESCRIPTION	COMMENTS
Common reference range		
Children	<2 ng/dL	Estradiol is most active of endogenous estrogens
Adult women, early cycle	1.8–2.4 ng/dL	
Adult women, midcycle	16.6–23.2 ng/dL	
Adult women, luteal phase	6.3–7.3 ng/dL	
Critical values	Not established	Extremely high or low values should be reported quickly
Inherent activity	Yes	Develops/maintains female reproductive system and feeds back to pituitary to regulate other hormone secretion
Location	Females: secreted by granulosa cells	
	Males: converted from testosterone and secreted from testes	
Causes of abnormal levels		
High	Estrogen-producing tumors, menstruation/preovulatory, 23rd to 41st wk of pregnancy	
Low	GnRH agonists	GnRH agonists monitored for females during treatment for precocious puberty
	Menopause, premature ovarian failure	
Signs and symptoms		
High level	N/A	
Low level	Hot flashes/night sweats	
After event, time until…	N/A	
Causes of spurious results	Radioactive pharmaceuticals and oral contraceptives	
Additional info	Used to monitor fertility	
	Estradiol >80 pg/mL on day 3 suggests adequate ovarian reserve	

Estrogen and Progesterone Receptors

PARAMETER	DESCRIPTION	COMMENTS
Common reference range	N/A	Not a normal serum laboratory value, only determined from breast biopsies
Critical value	N/A	
Inherent activity	Growth of breast and other hormone sensitive cells	
Location	Throughout the body (e.g., breast tissue, ovaries, bone)	
Causes of abnormal levels		
High	It is unknown if levels are higher in cancer, but checked to determine if blocking the receptors with hormonal therapy will be useful	
Low	N/A	
Signs and symptoms		
High level	N/A	
Low level	N/A	
After event, time until…	N/A	
Causes of spurious results	N/A	
Additional info	Lack of estrogen receptors is associated with a worse prognosis	Antiestrogens and aromatase inhibitors often given if these receptors are positive in women with breast cancer

Ethylene Glycol

PARAMETER	DESCRIPTION	COMMENTS
Common reference range	0 mg/dL	
Critical values	>20 mg/dL increases likelihood of toxicity	
Inherent activity	Metabolized to toxic metabolites (including aldehydes)	Used in suicide attempts and as an ethanol substitute
Location	Alimentary canal, blood, urine if ingested	
Causes of abnormal levels		
High	Antifreeze ingestion	
Low	N/A	
Signs and symptoms		
High level	CNS impairment/hallucinations, cardiotoxicity, nephrotoxicity, anion gap metabolic acidosis, osmolar gap, calcium oxalate crystalluria	
Low level	N/A	
After event, time until…	N/A	
Causes of spurious results	APAP and propylene glycol interact with older assay types	
Additional info	Results may not return in time to react	

Factor V Leiden

PARAMETER	DESCRIPTION	COMMENTS
Common reference range	Negative	Refers to PCR genetic test; APC clotting time assays are available and generally performed first
Critical values	Positive	
Inherent activity	Those with factor V Leiden mutation have resistance to APC-mediated factor V degradation	
Location	DNA	
Causes of abnormal levels		
High	Genetics	Not routinely monitored with any medications
Low	N/A	
Signs and symptoms		
High level	Thrombosis	
Low level	N/A	
After event, time until…	N/A	
Causes of spurious results	Direct thrombin inhibitors and lupus anticoagulant can cause positive APC clotting time results	
Additional info	Factor V Leiden is the most common genetic cause of VTE	

Ferritin

PARAMETER	DESCRIPTION	COMMENTS
Common reference range	>10–20 ng/mL	
Critical values	N/A	
Inherent activity	Ferritin is a storage form of iron	Serum levels are an indirect measure of iron stores
Location	Macrophages; but is also in plasma	
Causes of abnormal levels		
High	Iron overload	
	Inflammation/infection/fever	
Low	Iron deficiency (GI/GU bleed, inadequate consumption, IBD, pica)	
Signs and symptoms		
High level	Fever, infectious symptoms, inflammation (depends on cause), iron toxicity (CHF, cirrhosis, diabetes)	
Low level	Fatigue, pallor, tachycardia, numbness	
After event, time until…	N/A	
Causes of spurious results	Inflammation/infection/fever can mask iron deficiency anemia by increasing ferritin	Soluble transferrin receptor concentrations could be an alternative measure of iron deficiency
Additional info	N/A	

FEV$_1$ (Forced Expiratory Volume in 1 Second)

PARAMETER	DESCRIPTION	COMMENTS
Common reference range	>80% of predicted normal	
Critical values	<30% of predicted normal	
Inherent activity	N/A	Measures the volume of air expired forcefully in 1 sec
Location	N/A	
Causes of abnormal levels		
High	N/A	
Low	Asthma, COPD, idiopathic pulmonary fibrosis, sarcoidosis, pneumothorax, pleural effusions, morbid obesity, ascites	
Signs and symptoms		
High level	N/A	
Low level	Dyspnea, wheezing	
After event, time until…	N/A	
Causes of spurious results	Inactive reversible airway disease (false negative)	
Additional info	N/A	

FEV₁/FVC		
PARAMETER	DESCRIPTION	COMMENTS
Common reference range	>80%	
Critical values	N/A	
Inherent activity	N/A	
Location	N/A	
Causes of abnormal levels		
High	Idiopathic pulmonary fibrosis, sarcoidosis, pneumothorax, pleural effusions, morbid obesity, ascites	
Low	Airway obstruction or restriction (asthma, COPD)	
Signs and symptoms		
High level	Dependent on cause	
Low level	Dyspnea, wheezing, cough	
After event, time until…	N/A	
Causes of spurious results	N/A	
Additional info	Ratio <70% consistent with COPD; restrictive airway disease may present with normal FEV₁/FVC ratios as well	

Folate

PARAMETER	DESCRIPTION	COMMENTS
Common reference range	5–25 mcg/L	
Critical values	N/A	
Inherent activity	Necessary for DNA, amino acid, and neurotransmitter synthesis	
Location	Stored in liver	
Causes of abnormal levels		
High	N/A	
Low	Phenytoin, primidone, phenobarbital, methotrexate, oral contraceptives, pentamidine, sulfasalazine, sulfamethoxazole, triamterene, trimethoprim	Not routinely monitored with medications listed
	Inadequate dietary intake, ileal resection, gastrectomy, celiac sprue, alcoholics, pregnancy	Occurs after 4–5 mo of deficient diet
Signs and symptoms		
High level	N/A	
Low level	Loss of appetite, abnormalities of taste/smell, paresthesias, macrocytic anemia, memory impairment, spina bifida	
After event, time until…		
Initial elevation	Folate level restoration causes rapid symptomatic improvement but normal Hct levels may take 2 mo to attain	Event: folate supplementation
Causes of spurious results	N/A	
Additional info	Folate is also known as pteroylglutamic acid	

Fractional Excretion of Sodium (FENa)

PARAMETER	DESCRIPTION	COMMENTS
Common reference range	1% to 2%	Values between 1% and 2% do not help distinguish causes of acute kidney injury
Critical value	<1%	
	>2%	
Inherent activity	N/A	
Location		
Production/storage	N/A	
Secretion/excretion	Renal	
Causes of abnormal levels		
High	Renal tubular damage	
Low	Hypovolemia	
Signs and symptoms		
High level	N/A	
Low level	Dehydration	
After event, time until...		
Initial elevation	N/A	
Peak values	N/A	
Normalization	N/A	
Causes of spurious results	Acute diuretic use	May increase FE_{NA} to 20% or more; FEUrea recommended if recent diuretic use
Additional info	$FE_{Na} (\%) = \dfrac{Urine_{Na} / Serum_{Na}}{Urine_{Cr} / Serum_{Cr}} \times 100$	

Fractional Excretion of Urea (FEUrea)

PARAMETER	DESCRIPTION	COMMENTS
Common reference range	35% to 50%	
Critical value	<35%	
	>50%	
Inherent activity	N/A	
Location		
Production/storage	N/A	
Secretion/ excretion	Renal	
Causes of abnormal levels		
High	Renal tubular damage	
Low	Hypovolemia	
Signs and symptoms		
High level	N/A	
Low level	Dehydration	
After event, time until…		
Initial elevation	N/A	
Peak values	N/A	
Normalization	N/A	
Causes of spurious results	N/A	
Additional info	FEUrea recommended to evaluate cause of acute kidney injury if recent diuretic use	

Free T4 (Thyroxine)

PARAMETER	DESCRIPTION	COMMENTS
Common reference range	0.8–1.5 ng/dL	
Critical value	Not established	Extremely high or low values should be reported quickly
Inherent activity	Probably	Some influence on basal metabolic rate; T3 most active
Location		
Production	Thyroid gland	
Storage	Thyroid gland	Bound mostly to thyroglobulin
Secretion/excretion	From thyroid to blood	33% converted to T3 outside thyroid
Causes of abnormal levels		
High	T4 supplements	
	Hyperthyroidism	
Low	Hypothyroidism	
Signs and symptoms		
High level	Nervousness, weight loss, heat intolerance, tachycardia, diaphoresis	Signs and symptoms of hyperthyroidism
Low level	Lethargy, constipation, dry skin, cold intolerance, slow speech, confusion	Signs and symptoms of hypothyroidism
After event, time until…		
Initial elevation	Weeks to months	
Peak values	Weeks to months	Increases within hours in acute T4 overdose
Normalization	Same as onset	Assumes insult removed or effectively treated
Causes of spurious results	TGP abnormalities	Dependent on assay
Additional info	N/A	

T4 reference range
11.5 – 22.7 pmol/L
(at RIH)

Fructosamine

PARAMETER	DESCRIPTION	COMMENTS
Common reference range	<285 µmol/L	
Critical value	N/A	
Inherent activity	No	
Location		
Production	N/A	
Storage	N/A	
Secretion/ excretion	N/A	
Causes of abnormal levels		
High	Elevated glucose concentrations	Mostly seen in patients with diabetes
Low	Low albumin levels	
Signs and symptoms		
High level	Signs and symptoms of hyperglycemia	
Low level	N/A	
After event, time until…	N/A	
Causes of spurious results	Serum hemoglobin concentrations >100 mg/dL, serum bilirubin >4 mg/dL, serum ascorbic acid >5 mg/dL	Normally <15 mg/dL
Additional info	Correlates with glucose control over a 2–3 wk period	

FSH (Follicle Stimulating Hormone)

PARAMETER	DESCRIPTION	COMMENTS
Common reference range		
Children	5–10 million International Units/mL	Sometimes multiple blood specimens are necessary because of episodic increases of FSH
Adult women, early cycle and luteal phase	5–25 million International Units/mL	
Adult women, midcycle	20–30 million International Units/mL	
Menopausal women	40–250 million International Units/mL	
Critical values	N/A	Extreme values should be reported quickly
Inherent activity	Yes	Females: causes growth of ovarian follicles
Location	Produced/stored in anterior pituitary	
Causes of abnormal levels		
High	Phenytoin, dopamine agonists, cimetidine, GnRH, ketoconazole, naloxone, pravastatin, spironolactone, tamoxifen	Monitored with GnRH agonists
	Premature ovarian failure, menopause	Clomiphene challenge: compares FSH before and after clomiphene administration to determine ovarian reserve
Low	Danazol, carbamazepine, diethylstilbestrol, digoxin, estrogen, megestrol, phenothiazines, pravastatin, tamoxifen, testosterone	Not routinely monitored with mediations listed
	Ovarian tumors, pituitary adenoma, adrenal tumors, polycystic ovarian disease, eating disorders	
Signs and symptoms		
High level	Hot flashes/night sweats	
Low level	Virilization, galactorrhea/visual change, hirsutism/acne/obesity, cachexia/decreased BMI	Dependent on cause
After event, time until...	N/A	
Causes of spurious results	Recently administered radioisotopes, hemolysis of blood sample	
Additional info	FSH >10 million International Units/mL on day 3 suggests ovarian reserve	

G6PD (Glucose-6-Phosphate Dehydrogenase)

PARAMETER	DESCRIPTION	COMMENTS
Common reference range	Nondeficient	
Critical values	>90% deficient	Patients will have hemolytic crisis with oxidative medications
Inherent activity	Intracellular enzyme that produces glutathione	
Location	RBCs	
Causes of abnormal levels		
High	N/A	
Low	Genetic	
Signs and symptoms		
High level	N/A	
Low level	Oxidizing drugs (sulfonamides and ASA among others)/infection/ fava beans in patients with G6PD deficiency can cause hemolysis	
After event, time until…	N/A	
Causes of spurious results	N/A	
Additional info	G6PD deficiency is sometimes referred to as favism	

Galactomannan Assay

PARAMETER	DESCRIPTION	COMMENTS
Common reference range	Negative	
Critical value	Positive	Highly immunogenic component released by the fungal cell wall
Inherent activity	None	
Location		
Production	Fungal cell wall	
Storage	Serum	
Secretion/excretion	N/A	
Causes of abnormal levels		
High	Fungal infection with *Aspergillus*	
Low	N/A	
Signs and symptoms		
High level	Related to location of *Aspergillus* infection	
Low level	N/A	
After event, time until…		
Initial elevation	N/A	
Peak values	N/A	
Normalization	N/A	
Causes of spurious results	N/A	
Additional info	May be used to test body fluids such as blood, bronchioalveolar lavage fluid, urine, and cerebrospinal fluid; test is performed to use in conjunction with other diagnostic methods to support the diagnosis of invasive fungal infections	

Gamma-Glutamyl Transpeptidase (GGTP)

PARAMETER	DESCRIPTION	COMMENTS
Common reference range	1–94 units/L	
Critical value	N/A	
Inherent activity	Yes	Catalyzes the transfer of the gamma-glutamyl group from the gamma-glutamyl peptides to other peptides and amino acids
Location		
Production	Intracellular enzyme	
Storage	Liver, kidneys, pancreas, spleen, heart, brain and seminal vesicles	
Secretion/excretion	N/A	
Causes of abnormal levels		
High	Phenytoin, phenobarbital, carbamazepine, alcohol	Monitored if toxicity suspected
	Pancreatic disease, MI, severe chronic obstructive pulmonary disorders, SLE, hyperthyroidism, RA	Generally seen in diseases which affect liver, pancreas and biliary tract
Low	N/A	
Signs and symptoms		
High level	Varies with underlying disease	Reflects tissue or organ damage
Low level	N/A	
After event, time until…	N/A	
Causes of spurious results	N/A	
Additional info	N/A	

Haptoglobin

PARAMETER	DESCRIPTION	COMMENTS
Common reference range	30–200 mg/dL	Limited sensitivity and specificity (unless level is very low)
Critical values	N/A	
Inherent activity	Binds excess Hgb, acts as acute phase reactant	
Location	Produced in liver	
Causes of abnormal levels		
High	Biliary obstruction, nephrotic syndrome, inflammation/ infection/fever	
Low	Sulfonamides, nitrofurantoin, phenazopyridine, primaquine, dapsone in patients with G6PD	Haptoglobin not routinely monitored with medications listed
	Hemolysis	
Signs and symptoms		
High level	Abdominal pain, jaundice, peripheral edema (dependent on cause)	
Low level	Jaundice, discoloration of urine (brown), splenomegaly	
After event, time until…	N/A	
Causes of spurious results	Levels can be high/normal with hemolysis if patient is taking steroids	
Additional info	N/A	

Hemoglobin A1c

PARAMETER	DESCRIPTION	COMMENTS
Common reference range	4% to 6%	Represents average glucose levels past 2–3 mo
Critical value	N/A	
Inherent activity	Yes	Oxygen and glucose carrier
Location		
Production	Bone marrow	In newborns in liver and spleen
Storage	Not stored	Circulates in blood
Secretion/ excretion	Older RBCs removed by spleen	Transformed to bilirubin
Causes of abnormal levels		
High	Diabetes mellitus	
Low	N/A	
Signs and symptoms		
High level	Signs and symptoms of hyperglycemia	
Low level	N/A	
After event, time until…		
Initial elevation	2–4 mo	
Peak values	N/A	
Normalization	2–4 mo	
Causes of spurious results	Alcoholism, uremia, increased triglycerides, hemolysis, polycythemia	
Additional info	Fasting not required	

Hemoglobin (Hgb)/Hematocrit (Hct)

PARAMETER	DESCRIPTION		COMMENTS
Common reference range			
Adults	**Hgb** Males: 14–17.5 g/dL Females: 12.3–15.3 g/dL **Hct** Males: 42% to 50% Females: 36% to 45%		Commonly only one of these lab values is mentioned because they provide similar information and are commonly related by a factor of 3 (except if RBC size/shape abnormality)
Pediatrics	**Hgb**	**Hct**	
1–3 days old	18.5 g/dL	56%	
1 wk old	17.5 g/dL	54%	
2 wk old	16.5 g/dL	51%	
1 mo old	14.0 g/dL	43%	
2 mo old	11.5 g/dL	35%	
3–6 mo old	11.5 g/dL	35%	
0.5–2 yr old	12.0 g/dL	36%	
2–6 yr old	12.5 g/dL	37%	
6–12 yr old	13.5 g/dL	40%	
12–18 yr old			
Males	14.5 g/dL	43%	
Females	14.0 g/dL	41%	
Critical values	Hgb <7 g/dL, <8–9 g/dL if cardiac disease		Transfusion recommended Decrease dose/hold ESA
	>12 g/dL if on ESA Hct >50%		Poor outcomes associated in polycythemia vera
Inherent activity	Hgb: delivers O_2 to tissues Hct: N/A		Hct is the percent volume of blood that is composed of RBCs
Location	Hgb: RBCs		
Causes of abnormal levels			
High	ESAs, androgens		Monitor Hgb q 1–2 wk initially, then every month for ESAs
	Polycythemia (e.g., as a result from hypoxia), renal artery stenosis, high altitude		
Low	Anticoagulants/antiplatelets, chemotherapy, antibiotics, zidovudine		Monitoring dependent on medication (therapeutic anticoagulation daily initially vs. antiplatelets periodically)
	Under production (e.g., due to deficiency of factors involved like iron, folate or vit B_{12}), loss of blood (can occur occultly), premature RBC destruction (e.g., hemolytic anemia)		

(continued)

Hemoglobin (Hgb)/Hematocrit (Hct) (Cont.)

Signs and symptoms		
High level	Dependent on cause	
Low level	Fatigue, pallor, bleeding	
After event, time until…		
Normalization	Commonly takes 6–8 wk to return levels to normal (depending on disease process/resolution)	Event: anemia
Causes of spurious results	IV fluid administration can lower Hgb/Hct and give the appearance of acute blood loss	
Additional info	N/A	

Heparin-Induced Platelet Antibodies

PARAMETER	DESCRIPTION	COMMENTS
Common reference range	Negative	Assay is sensitive but not specific
Critical values	Positive	
Inherent activity	Bind to heparin/PF4 complex causing aggregation/removal of platelets and thrombin formation	
Location	Blood	
Causes of abnormal levels		
High	Heparin exposure (more common with UFH than LMWH)	Not routinely monitored with UFH/LMWH unless HIT suspected
Low	N/A	
Signs and symptoms		
High level	Thrombosis (venous and arterial), skin lesions, chills/cardiorespiratory distress after UFH bolus	
Low level	N/A	
After event, time until...	N/A	
Causes of spurious results	HD patients may have false positive results	
Additional info	Commonly ordered when platelets decrease by 50% (especially if 4T test suggests high likelihood of HIT); this test is an ELISA test that generally requires confirmation with a more specific assay (e.g., SRA)	Commonly, platelets decrease 5–14 days after heparin but can decrease in 1 day if previous exposure

High Density Lipoprotein (HDL)

PARAMETER	DESCRIPTION	COMMENTS
Common reference range	Low: <40 mg/dL High: >60 mg/dL	
Critical value	None established	
Inherent activity	Yes	Removes cholesterol from atherosclerotic plaques in arteries
Location		
Production	Intestines and liver	
Storage	Serum	
Secretion/excretion	Bile	
Causes of abnormal levels		
High	Estrogens, nicotinic acid, HMG-COA reductase inhibitors, omega-3 fatty acids	
Low	Beta-blockers, danazol, isotretinoin, progestins, protease inhibitors	Danazol, isotretinoin, protease inhibitors, are commonly monitored
	Familial hypoalphalipoproteinemia, DM, hypothyroidism, nephrotic syndrome, obesity, sedentary lifestyle	
Signs and symptoms		
High level	N/A	
Low level	Related to underlying cause	
After event, time until…		
Initial elevation	Days to weeks	
Peak values	Days to weeks	
Normalization	Weeks to months	Assumes appropriate treatment
Causes of spurious results	Nonfasting state	
Additional info	Considered a negative risk factor for CHD if elevated	

HIV Antibody Test

PARAMETER	DESCRIPTION	COMMENTS
Common reference range	Nonreactive (negative)	
Critical value	Reactive (positive)	
Inherent activity	None	
Location		
Production	N/A	
Storage	Serum	
Secretion/ excretion	N/A	
Causes of abnormal levels		
High	HIV infection	
Low	N/A	
Signs and symptoms		
High level	Dependent on HIV progression	
Low level	N/A	
After event, time until…		
Initial elevation	4–8 wk after exposure to the virus	May take up to 6–12 mo in some patients
Peak values	N/A	
Normalization	N/A	
Causes of spurious results	Reactivity of antibodies to human leukocyte antigen (HLA), autoimmune diseases, recent influenza vaccination, acute viral infection, alcoholic liver disease, chronic renal failure requiring hemodialysis, lymphoma, hematologic malignancies, rapid plasma reagin positive serum, and improper specimen handling	False positives
	Immunosuppressive therapy, severe hypogammaglobulinemia, and testing when HIV antibody production is too low (too early [first 1–2 wk after infection] or too late in the course of HIV infection)	False negatives
Additional info	Sensitivity and specificity of about 99%; however, a positive test must be confirmed with a more specific test such as the Western blot	

HIV DNA PCR

PARAMETER	DESCRIPTION	COMMENTS
Common reference range	Negative	Negative tests at birth should be repeated at 14 days of life since the assay sensitivity is increased by 2 wk of life
Critical value	Positive	In order to confirm the diagnosis of HIV infection, a positive result at any sampling time needs to be confirmed by a second HIV virologic test
Inherent activity	N/A	
Location		
Production	N/A	
Storage	Peripheral blood mononuclear cells (PBMCs)	
Secretion/excretion	N/A	
Causes of abnormal levels		
High	HIV infection	
Low	N/A	
Signs and symptoms		
High level	N/A	
Low level	N/A	
After event, time until...		
Initial elevation	Birth to 14 days old	Test should be repeated at 1–2 mo and age 3–6 mo
Peak values	N/A	
Normalization	N/A	
Causes of spurious results		
Additional info	HIV infection may be excluded in infants with two or more negative HIV virologic results when initial testing occurred at age ≥1 mo and the second testing occurred at age ≥4 mo	Recommended for the diagnosis of HIV infection in infants (<18 mo of age) born to HIV-infected mothers Antibody tests are not useful for diagnosing HIV infection in infants since maternal HIV antibodies can persist in the infant for up to 18 mo after birth

HIV RNA Concentration (Viral Load)

PARAMETER	DESCRIPTION	COMMENTS
Common reference range	Undetectable	
Critical value	>100,000 HIV copies/mL	Also known as HIV viral load
Inherent activity	None	
Location		
Production	N/A	
Storage	Serum	
Secretion/ excretion	N/A	
Causes of abnormal levels		
High	Progressive HIV infection	
Low	Antiretroviral therapy	
Signs and symptoms		
High level	Dependent on HIV progression	
Low level	N/A	
After event, time until…		
Initial elevation	N/A	
Peak values	N/A	
Normalization	16–24 wk	Patients should achieve an undetectable VL in 16–24 wk after initiating antiretroviral therapy
Causes of spurious results	Recent vaccination	HIV RNA testing not recommended during these periods as viral may increase for 2–4 wk
	Acute illness	
Additional info	Also known as the HIV viral load or the marker of patients virologic status	
	Essential component of the management of patients with HIV-1 infection	
	Used in conjunction with the CD4+ T lymphocyte count to provide essential information regarding the patients' immunologic and virologic status, risk of disease progression to AIDS, and whether to initiate or change antiretroviral therapy	

HIV Western Blot

PARAMETER	DESCRIPTION	COMMENTS
Common reference range	Negative	Results are classified as positive, negative, or indeterminate
Critical value	Positive	Positive if bands for two of the three HIV specific proteins (p24, gp41, gp120/160)
Inherent activity	N/A	
Location		
Production	N/A	
Storage	Serum	
Secretion/ excretion	N/A	
Causes of abnormal levels		
High	HIV infection	
Low	N/A	
Signs and symptoms		
High level	Dependent on HIV progression	
Low level	N/A	
After event, time until...		
Initial elevation	4–8 wk after exposure to the virus	May take up to 6–12 mo in some patients
Peak values	N/A	
Normalization	N/A	
Causes of spurious results	Testing too early or too late in the course of HIV infection, cross-reactivity with HIV-2 infection, cross-reactivity with HIV-1 subtype O, or the production of nonspecific antibody reactions	Indeterminate results
Additional info	Should be used as a confirmatory test for HIV after a positive HIV antibody test	
	Not to be used as an initial screen for HIV as many tests result as indeterminate, it is technically difficult to perform, and expensive	
	Test results take approximately 1–2 wk for results	

HLA-B* 5701

PARAMETER	DESCRIPTION	COMMENTS
Common reference range	Negative	
Critical value	Positive	Abacavir should be avoided in patients with a positive result
Inherent activity	N/A	
Location		
Production	N/A	
Storage	MHC class I	
Secretion/excretion	N/A	
Causes of abnormal levels		
High	Presence of HLA-B* 5701 allele	
Low	N/A	
Signs and symptoms		
High level	Possible hypersensitivity reaction	Presence of the MHC class I allele HLA-B*5701 indicates patients are at risk of developing a life-threatening hypersensitivity reaction to the antiretroviral abacavir
Low level	N/A	
After event, time until...		
Initial elevation	N/A	
Peak values	N/A	
Normalization	N/A	
Causes of spurious results	N/A	
Additional info	Test should be performed prior to the initiation of abacavir	

Homocysteine

PARAMETER	DESCRIPTION	COMMENTS
Common reference range	5–15 µmol/L	Dependent on institution/methods
Critical values	N/A	
Inherent activity	Precursor to methionine, degrades components of vasculature and is associated with increased cardiovascular risk	
Location	Serum	
Causes of abnormal levels		
High	B6, B12, folate deficiency (see B12 and folate monograph for specifics)	
Low	N/A	
Signs and symptoms		
High level	See B12 and folate monograph for specifics	
Low level	N/A	
After event, time until…	N/A	
Causes of spurious results	Hypothyroidism, renal failure	
Additional info	N/A	

Human Chorionic Gonadotropin (hCG)

PARAMETER	DESCRIPTION	COMMENTS
Common reference range	<5 million International Units/mL	Beta subunit commonly measured, serum levels drawn when used as a tumor marker; pediatric range unknown
Critical value	N/A	If elevated in males or in nonpregnant females, cancer is suspected
Inherent activity	Promotes luteal progesterone production	
Location	Produced by cells that make up the placenta	Detected in patient serum and urine
Causes of abnormal levels		
High	Pregnancy, testicular cancer, germ cell tumors, increased in other rare tumors	
Low	N/A	
Signs and symptoms		
High level	N/A	
Low level	N/A	
After event, time until…	N/A	
Causes of spurious results	For pregnancy, if tested too soon (<10 days) after menses	
Additional info	Routinely used to test pregnancy (levels >25 are consistent with pregnancy and should double every 2–3 days); qualitative tests more sensitive than quantitative tests; used to monitor response to oncologic therapy during/after treatment	Levels >50,000 million International Units/mL are associated with poor prognosis for nonseminomatous disease

Human Epidermal Growth Factor Receptor 2 (HER-2)

PARAMETER	DESCRIPTION	COMMENTS
Common reference range	Considered positive by IHC if 3+ cells stain for HER-2 or by FISH if HER-2 gene copy number >6 or FISH ratio >2.2	Not a normal serum laboratory value, only determined in breast biopsies
Critical value	N/A	
Inherent activity	Protein involved in normal growth and development of cells by activating intracellular pathways that send growth signals to the nucleus	In cancer the growth signal is abnormal and amplified leading to uncontrolled proliferation of the cancerous cells
Location	Surface of many epidermal cells	
Causes of abnormal levels		
High	Cancer (either number of receptors may be higher or there may be an increase in HER-2 gene copies indicating increased function of the gene)	
Low	N/A	
Signs and symptoms		
High level	N/A	
Low level	N/A	
After event, time until…	N/A	
Causes of spurious results	N/A	
Additional info	Anti-HER-2 therapies often given if positive	

INR/PT (International Normalized Ratio and Prothrombin Time)

PARAMETER	DESCRIPTION	COMMENTS
Common reference range	INR <1.2 (in general population, commonly 2–3 or 2.5–3.5 if taking warfarin) PT 10–13 sec	Desired INR ranges will vary if patient is on warfarin and depending on indication for warfarin
Critical value	INR: lower limit critical values depend on indication >5 while on warfarin suggests need to modify therapy and possibly administer low dose oral vitamin K	
Inherent activity	N/A	Indirect measure of coagulation factors
Location		
Production	Coagulation factors produced in liver	
Causes of abnormal levels		
High	Warfarin	Warfarin should be monitored
	Liver disease, pyrexia, DIC, primary fibrinolysis, malabsorption/malnutrition	
Low	Vitamin K (if taking warfarin)	
Signs and symptoms		
High level	Increased risk of bleeding and ecchymosis	Risk increases as INR/PT increases
Low level	Thrombosis if predisposed	
After event, time until…		
Initial elevation	~48 hr (variable)	Event: warfarin initiation
Peak values	5–7 days (variable)	
Normalization	Hours to days	Variable if reversed with FFP/vitamin K/holding warfarin
Causes of spurious results	Improper laboratory collection (e.g., from central venous catheter in patients with HD)	
Additional info	INR = (patient PT/control PT)[ISI]	

Iron

PARAMETER	DESCRIPTION	COMMENTS
Common reference range	50–150 mcg/dL	
Critical values	N/A	
Inherent activity	Iron is used in Hgb synthesis and energy metabolism	Measures iron bound to transferrin
Location	RBCs, bone marrow, reticuloendothelial system	
Causes of abnormal levels		
High	Iron overload, hemolytic anemia	Intermittently assessed with iron therapy
Low	Acid suppressive therapies, tetracyclines, polyvalent cationic antacids	Not commonly monitored with medications listed
	Iron deficiency (GI/GU bleed, inadequate consumption, IBD, pica), malignancy, infection, uremia	
Signs and symptoms		
High level	Iron toxicity (CHF, cirrhosis, diabetes)	
Low level	Fatigue, pallor, tachycardia, numbness, fever, infectious symptoms, inflammation (depends on cause)	
After event, time until…	N/A	
Causes of spurious results	N/A	
Additional info	Ferritin more useful to assess iron deficiency anemia due to false negatives associated with serum iron	

Lactate (Lactic Acid)

PARAMETER	DESCRIPTION	COMMENTS
Common reference range	0.6–2.2 mEq/L (venous) 0.3–0.8 mEq/L (arterial)	Arterial blood sample is preferred
Critical values	>4 mEq/L	
Inherent activity	A breakdown product of anaerobic metabolism	
Location	Various tissues including muscle	
Causes of abnormal levels		
High	Ethanol, ethylene glycol, methanol, nitroprusside, salicylates, parenteral lorazepam, zidovudine, possibly metformin (if impaired kidney function)	Monitored in situations of overdose/suspected toxicity and when suspected clinically
	Exercise, MI/arrhythmia, rhabdomyolysis, diabetes, liver/kidney failure, shock, hypoxia	
Low	N/A	
Signs and symptoms		
High level	Weakness, hyperventilation, mental status changes, coma, death	
Low level	N/A	
After event, time until…	N/A	
Causes of spurious results	N/A	
Additional info	Causes an anion gap acidosis	

LDH (Lactic Acid Dehydrogenase)

PARAMETER	DESCRIPTION	COMMENTS
Common reference range	100–210 International Units/L	Not specific when assessing MI
Critical values	N/A	
Inherent activity	Catalyzes lactate conversion to pyruvate	
Location	Heart, liver, lungs, kidneys, skeletal muscle, RBCs, lymphocytes	
Causes of abnormal levels		
High	MI, hemolysis, infection, liver/kidney disease	
Low	N/A	
Signs and symptoms		
High level	Dependent on cause	
Low level	N/A	
After event, time until…		
Initial elevation	24–48 hr	Event: MI
Peak values	2–3 days	
Normalization	8–14 days	
Causes of spurious results	Accidental hemolysis of sample	
Additional info	Composed of five isoenzymes (LDH1-5); commonly ordered in addition to other tests to assess hemolysis	

LH (Luteinizing Hormone)

PARAMETER	DESCRIPTION	COMMENTS
Common reference range		
Children	5–10 million International Units/mL	Often measured with FSH to determine hormonally-related functions/disorders
Adult women, early cycle and luteal phase	5–25 million International Units/mL	
Adult women, midcycle	40–80 million International Units/mL	
Menopausal women	>75 million International Units/mL	
Critical values	Not established	Extremely high or low values should be reported quickly
Inherent activity	Yes	Surge of LH prompts ovulation and production of progesterone
Location	Produced/stored in anterior pituitary	
Causes of abnormal levels		
High	Phenytoin, dopamine agonists, clomiphene, GnRH, GHRH, ketoconazole, mestranol, spironolactone	GnRH agonists, clomiphene monitored
	Premature ovarian failure, menopause, polycystic ovarian disease	
Low	Danazol, carbamazepine, CRH, diethylstilbestrol, digoxin, estrogen, megestrol, phenothiazines, pravastatin, progesterone, tamoxifen, testosterone	
	Pituitary adenoma, eating disorders	
Signs and symptoms		
High level	Hot flashes/night sweats, hirsutism/acne/obesity	Dependent on cause LH/FSH ratio >3
Low level	Galactorrhea/visual changes, cachexia/low BMI	Dependent on cause
After event, time until…	N/A	
Causes of spurious results	Recently administered radioisotopes, hemolysis of blood sample, pregnancy	
Additional info	N/A	

Lidocaine

PARAMETER	DESCRIPTION	COMMENTS
Common reference range	1.5–5 mg/L	Level can be drawn any time after steady state is reached (administered as infusion)
Critical values	>6 mg/L	
Inherent activity	Decreases neuronal sodium permeability	
Location	N/A	
Causes of abnormal levels		
High	Decreased clearance: liver disease, CHF, advanced age, propranolol, cimetidine	Commonly monitored if prolonged infusion or suspected toxicity
Low	N/A	
Signs and symptoms		
High level	>3 mg/L: drowsiness, dizziness, euphoria, paresthesias	
	>6 mg/L: muscle twitching, confusion, agitation, psychoses	
	>8 mg/L: CV depression, AV block, hypotension, seizures, coma, death	
Low level	N/A	
After event, time until…		
Normalization	Up to 24 hr to reach steady state	
Causes of spurious results	Disease states (including MI) causing elevated levels of alpha-1-acid glycoprotein may require higher levels to exert desired effect	
Additional info	Active metabolite accumulates in renal failure	

Lipase

PARAMETER	DESCRIPTION	COMMENTS
Common reference range	<160 units/L	
Critical value	3–5 times the upper limit of normal	
Inherent activity	Yes	Catalyzes the hydrolysis of triglycerides into fatty acids and glycerol
Location		
Production	Pancreas	
Storage	Tongue, esophagus, stomach, small intestine, leukocytes, adipose tissue, lung, breast milk, liver	
Secretion/ excretion	Kidney	
Causes of abnormal levels		
High	Pancreatitis, ruptured abdominal aortic aneurysm, intestinal infarction, renal failure, nephrolithiasis, diabetic ketoacidosis, alcoholism	
Low	N/A	
Signs and symptoms		
High level	Related to underlying disorder	
Low level	N/A	
After event, time until…		
Initial elevation	2–6 hr	
Peak values	12–30 hr	
Normalization	8–14 days	Half-life of 7–14 hr
Causes of spurious results	N/A	
Additional info	May have superior specificity for pancreatitis as compared to amylase	

Lithium

PARAMETER	DESCRIPTION	COMMENTS
Common reference range	Acute: 0.5–1.2 mEq/L	Level recommended 12 hr after evening dose
	Maintenance: 0.6–0.8 mEq/L	
Critical values	>2 mEq/L	
Inherent activity	Mood stabilizing effects	
Location	N/A	
Causes of abnormal levels		
High	Thiazide diuretics, ACEIs, renal impairment	Levels commonly monitored for efficacy/safety
Low	N/A	
Signs and symptoms		
High level	>1.5 mEq/L associated with fine tremors, GI disturbances, muscle weakness, polyuria, and polydipsia	
	>2.5 mEq/L associated with coarse tremors, confusion, delirium, slurred speech and vomiting	
	>3.5 mEq/L seizures, coma, and death	
Low level	N/A	
After event, time until…		
Normalization	Up to 1 wk until steady state	
Causes of spurious results	Hemolysis can artificially elevate level	
	Carbamazepine, quinidine, procainamide, N-acetylprocainamide, lidocaine, and valproic acid interfere with ion selective electrode assay	
Additional info	N/A	

Low Density Lipoprotein (LDL)

PARAMETER	DESCRIPTION	COMMENTS
Common reference range	Optimal: <100 mg/dL Near optimal: 100–129 mg/dL Borderline high: 130–159 mg/dL High: 160–189 mg/dL Very high: ≥190 mg/dL	Must be measured in fasting state; <70 mg/dL considered optimal if high risk (e.g., CAD + DM)
Critical value	>190 mg/dL	
Inherent activity	Yes	Major carrier of cholesterol
Location		
Production	Liver	
Storage	Serum	
Secretion/ excretion	Bile	
Causes of abnormal levels		
High	Corticosteroids, cyclosporine, danazol, isotretinoin, progestins, thiazides diuretics	LDL monitoring advised with danazol, and isotretinoin
	Familial hypercholesterolemia, DM, hypothyroidism, nephrotic syndrome, obesity, sedentary lifestyle	
Low	HMG-COA reductase inhibitors, nicotinic acid, bile acid sequestrants, ezetimibe	Medications listed are commonly monitored
	Severe hepatic disease	
Signs and symptoms		
High level	Signs/symptoms consistent with atherosclerotic disease	
Low level	N/A	
After event, time until…		
Initial elevation	Days to weeks	
Peak values	Days to weeks	
Normalization	Weeks to months	Assumes appropriate treatment
Causes of spurious results	Nonfasting state	
Additional info	Elevated LDL is risk factor for CHD	

Lymphocytes

PARAMETER	DESCRIPTION	COMMENTS
Common reference range	20% to 40 %	
Critical value	>4000 cells/μL	
	<1000 cells/μL	
Inherent activity	Yes	Involved in cell mediated immunity
Location		
Production	Bone marrow	
Storage	Thymus	T lymphocytes mature in thymus
	Bone marrow	B lymphocytes mature in bone marrow
	Serum	
Secretion/ excretion	N/A	
Causes of abnormal levels		
High	Infectious mononucleosis	Rubella, varicella, mumps, CMV
	Viral infections	
	Pertussis	
	Tuberculosis	
	Syphilis	
	Lymphoma	
Low	Glucocorticoids	Hodgkin's disease
	HIV type 1	
	Radiation exposure	
	Lymphoma	
	Aplastic anemia	
Signs and symptoms		
High level	Related to underlying cause	
Low level	Related to underlying cause	
After event, time until…		
Initial elevation	N/A	
Peak values	N/A	
Normalization	N/A	
Causes of spurious results	N/A	
Additional info	N/A	

Lysergic Acid Diethylamide (LSD) (Urine Drug Screen)

PARAMETER	DESCRIPTION	COMMENTS
Common reference range	Negative	
Critical value	Positive	
Inherent activity	Yes	
Location		
Production	N/A	
Storage	N/A	
Secretion/excretion	N/A	
Causes of abnormal levels		
High	Ingestion, ocular instillation, buccal cavity placement of LSD	
Low	N/A	
Signs and symptoms		
High level	Unpredictable hallucinogenic effects, mydriasis, hyperthermia, tachycardia, hypertension, sweating, loss of appetite, sleeplessness, dry mouth, tremors	Flash-backs months later are possible
Low level	N/A	
After event, time until...		
Negative result	24–48 hr, typically	Up to 120 hr possible
Causes of spurious results	N/A	
Additional info	Schedule I drug with no legitimate medical use	

Magnesium

PARAMETER	DESCRIPTION	COMMENTS
Common reference range		
Adults	1.5–2.2 mEq/L (0.75–1.1 mmol/L)	
Newborns (0–6 days old)	1.2–2.6 mg/dL (0.6–1.3 mmol/L)	
Infants (7 days to 2 yr old)	1.6–2.6 mg/dL (0.8–1.3 mmol/L)	
Children (2–14 yr old)	1.5–2.3 mg/dL (0.75–1.15 mmol/L)	
Critical value	>5 or <1 mEq/L (>2.5 or <0.5 mmol/L)	Acute changes more dangerous than chronic abnormalities
Inherent activity	Yes	Enzyme cofactor, thermoregulation, muscle contraction, nerve conduction, calcium and potassium homeostasis
Location		
Storage	50% bone, 45% intracellular fluid, 5% extracellular fluid	
Secretion/ excretion	Filtration by kidneys	3% to 5% reabsorbed
Causes of abnormal levels		
High	Renal failure (usually in presence of increased intake)	
Low	Diuretics, PPIs	Listed drugs should be monitored occasionally
	Excessive loss from GI tract or kidneys, decreased intake, alcoholism, pancreatitis	
Signs and symptoms		
High level	2–5 mEq/L: bradycardia, flushing, sweating, N/V, decreased clotting mechanisms	
	6 mEq/L: drowsiness, depressed reflexes	
	10–15 mEq/L: flaccid paralysis and increased PR and QT interval	
	>15 mEq/L: respiratory distress/ asystole	
Low level	Neuromuscular and cardiovascular manifestations including weakness, muscle fasciculations, tremor, tetany, increased reflexes, and ECG abnormalities	More severe with acute changes

(continued)

Magnesium (Cont.)

After event, time until…

Initial elevation	Variable	Faster change is more dangerous
Peak values	Variable	
Normalization	Days, if renal function is normal	Faster with appropriate treatment
Causes of spurious results	Hemolyzed samples (falsely elevated)	
Additional info	Hypomagnesemia commonly present with K and Ca deficiencies	

Manganese

PARAMETER	DESCRIPTION	COMMENTS
Common reference range		
Adults	Unknown normal range	
Pediatrics	2–3 mcg/L (36–55 µmol/L)	
	2.4–9.6 mcg/L (44–175 µmol/L)	Newborn
	0.8–2.1 mcg/L (15–38 µmol/L)	2–18 yr
Critical value	N/A	
Inherent activity	Yes	Enzyme cofactor; carbohydrate, protein, and lipid metabolism; protection of cells from free radicals; steroid biosynthesis; metabolism of biogenic amines; normal brain function
		Magnesium may substitute for manganese in most instances
Location		
Storage	Bone, liver, pancreas, pituitary gland, brain	Circulating manganese loosely bound to transmanganin
Secretion/ excretion	Primarily in biliary and pancreatic secretions; limited excretion in urine	Other GI routes also may be used in manganese overload
Causes of abnormal levels		
High	Manganese supplements, possibly during chronic TPN	Serum manganese concentration not routinely monitored
	Primarily through inhalation of manganese compounds, such as in manganese mines	
Low	After several months of deliberate omission from diet	
Signs and symptoms		
High level	Encephalopathy and profound neurological disturbances mimicking Parkinson's disease	Accumulates in liver and brain
		One of least toxic trace elements
Low level	Weight loss, slow hair and nail growth, hair color change, transient dermatitis, hypocholesterolemia, hypotriglyceridemia	Seen mostly in experimental subjects
After event, time until…	N/A	
Causes of spurious results	N/A	
Additional info	N/A	

Mantoux Test

PARAMETER	DESCRIPTION	COMMENTS
Common reference range	0 mm	Administered as an intradermal injection and is measured by the diameter of induration
Critical value	≥5 mm	≥5 mm: positive in persons at high risk of developing tuberculosis
	≥10 mm	≥10 mm: positive in patients who are not immunocompromised and possess no other risk factors for developing tuberculosis
	≥15 mm	≥15 mm: positive in persons at low risk for developing active infection with tuberculosis
Inherent activity	None	
Location		
Production	N/A	
Storage	N/A	
Secretion/ excretion	N/A	
Causes of abnormal levels		
High	Tuberculosis exposure	
Low	N/A	
Signs and symptoms		
High level	Fever, chills, night sweats, hemoptysis	
Low level	N/A	
After event, time until…		
Initial elevation	48–72 hr	
Peak values	N/A	
Normalization	N/A	
Causes of spurious results	TB vaccination	
Additional info	Available for the detection of latent TB	

Mean Corpuscular Hemoglobin Concentration (MCHC)

PARAMETER	DESCRIPTION	COMMENTS
Common reference range	33.4–35.5 g/dL	Normal values: normochromic Low values: hypochromic
Critical values	N/A	
Inherent activity	Hgb delivers oxygen to tissues	Estimates Hgb per RBC (controls for RBC size variation)
Location	RBCs	
Causes of abnormal levels		
High	N/A	Monitored to help identify cause of anemia
Low	Seen most often in iron deficiency	
Signs and symptoms		
High level	N/A	
Low level	Fatigue, pallor, bleeding	
After event, time until…	N/A	
Causes of spurious results	False elevation in hyperlipidemia	
Additional info	MCHC = Hgb/Hct	

Mean Corpuscular Hgb (MCH)

PARAMETER	DESCRIPTION	COMMENTS
Common reference range	27.5–33.2 pg/cell	
Critical values	N/A	
Inherent activity	Hgb delivers oxygen to tissues	
Location	RBCs	Estimates Hgb per RBC
Causes of abnormal levels		
High	B$_{12}$/folate deficiency, alcoholism, (see folate and B12 monographs for individual causes)	Monitored to help identify cause of anemia
Low	Iron deficiency, chronic disease	
Signs and symptoms		
High level	B$_{12}$/folate deficiency can cause neuropathies, loss of appetite/taste	
Low level	Fatigue, pallor, bleeding	
After event, time until…	N/A	
Causes of spurious results	Can be falsely elevated in hyperlipidemia	
Additional info	MCH = Hgb/RBC	

Mean Corpuscular Volume

PARAMETER	DESCRIPTION	COMMENTS
Common reference range	80–96 fL/cell	<80 indicates microcytosis >100 indicates macrocytosis
Critical values	N/A	
Inherent activity	N/A	A measure of RBC volume
Location	N/A	
Causes of abnormal levels		
High	B_{12}/folate deficiency, alcoholism (see folate and B12 monographs for individual causes)	Monitored to help identify cause of anemia
Low	Iron deficiency, chronic disease	
Signs and symptoms		
High level	B_{12}/folate deficiency can cause neuropathies, loss of appetite/taste	
Low level	Fatigue, pallor, bleeding	
After event, time until…	N/A	
Causes of spurious results	Reticulocytosis and hyperglycemia can cause a "false" elevation of MCV	
Additional info	N/A	

Methanol

PARAMETER	DESCRIPTION	COMMENTS
Common reference range	<0.05 mg/dL	
Critical values	>20 mg/dL CNS symptoms	
	>50 ocular toxicity	
Inherent activity	Metabolized to formaldehyde and formic acid	
Location	Concentrates in liver, kidney and eye	
Causes of abnormal levels		
High	Methanol ingestion	
Low	N/A	
Signs and symptoms		
High level	CNS depression, visual changes/blindness, N/V, anion gap metabolic acidosis, osmolar gap (but can also be normal)	
Low level	N/A	
After event, time until…		
Peak values	60 min	Event: methanol ingestion
Normalization	Variable, half-life is 15–30 hr	
Causes of spurious results	N/A	
Additional info	N/A	

Methylmalonate

PARAMETER	DESCRIPTION	COMMENTS
Common reference range	<300 nmol/L	Dependent on institution
Critical values	N/A	
Inherent activity	Precursor to succinic acid	
Location	Serum, urine	
Causes of abnormal levels		
High	B12 deficiency (see B12 monograph for specifics)	
Low	N/A	
Signs and symptoms		
High level	Loss of appetite, abnormalities of taste/smell, paresthesias, macrocytic anemia, memory impairment	
Low level	N/A	
After event, time until…	N/A	
Causes of spurious results	Renal impairment causes false elevations	
Additional info	Used to confirm B12 deficiency when B12 results equivocal or normal despite symptoms	

Monocytes

PARAMETER	DESCRIPTION	COMMENTS
Common reference range	2% to 8%	
Critical value	>800 cells/µL	
Inherent activity	Yes	Attack foreign cells
		Destruction of old erythrocytes, plasma lipids, denatured plasma proteins
Location		
Production	Bone marrow	
Storage	Lymph nodes, alveoli of the lungs, spleen, liver, bone marrow	
Secretion/ excretion	N/A	
Causes of abnormal levels		
High	Recovery state of acute bacterial infection, tuberculosis (disseminated), endocarditis, protozoal or rickettsial infection, leukemia	
Low	N/A	
Signs and symptoms		
High level	Related to underlying cause	
Low level	N/A	
After event, time until…		
Initial elevation	N/A	
Peak values	N/A	
Normalization	N/A	
Causes of spurious results	N/A	
Additional info	N/A	

Mycophenolic Acid

PARAMETER	DESCRIPTION	COMMENTS
Common reference range	Trough: 2.5–4 mg/L AUC: 30–60 mg × hr/L	AUC estimation requires trough, 30 min, and 120 min postdose levels
Critical values	N/A	
Inherent activity	Immunosuppressant	
Location	N/A	
Causes of abnormal levels		
High	Diminished glucuronidation capacity, metabolites may accumulate in renal impairment	Not routinely monitored unless toxicity suspected
Low	Antacids, bile acid sequestrants	
	Low albumin states and drug displacement interactions may cause falsely low total levels	
Signs and symptoms		
High level	Constipation, N/V/D, leukopenia	
Low level	Organ rejection	
After event, time until…	Approx. 3 days until steady state	
Causes of spurious results	Protein binding interactions	Unbound levels recommended in patients with suspected protein interactions
Additional info	Metabolite interacts with EMIT® method yielding higher levels than HPLC	

O$_2$ Saturation

PARAMETER	DESCRIPTION	COMMENTS
Common reference range	>95% (pulse oximetry)	Can be measured in arterial blood sample or with pulse oximetry (clip placed on finger and measures saturation with light)
Critical values	<90%	
Inherent activity	Measures Hgb O$_2$ saturation	
Location	Blood	
Causes of abnormal levels		
High	Excess O$_2$ administration	Commonly measured in hospital and periodically in patients with respiratory diseases
Low	Hypoventilation, high altitude, ventilation/perfusion mismatch	
Signs and symptoms		
High level	Alveolar edema/hemorrhage, diminished lung compliance	
Low level	Hyperventilation (if disease process impairs gas exchange), cyanosis, mental status changes, seizures, coma	
After event, time until…	N/A	
Causes of spurious results	Nail polish	
	Smokers and patients with hyperbilirubinemia may have falsely elevated pulse oximetry readings	
	Methylene blue can falsely decrease readings	
Additional info	N/A	

Opiates (Urine Drug Screen)

PARAMETER	DESCRIPTION	COMMENTS
Common reference range	Negative	
Critical value	Positive	Heroin use is confirmed by the presence of 6-acetylmorphine
Inherent activity	Yes	
Location		
Production/storage	N/A	
Secretion/excretion	Renal	
Causes of abnormal levels		
High	Ingestion, injection, dermal application, rectal insertion	
Low	N/A	
Signs and symptoms		
High level	CNS depression, miosis, drowsiness, constipation, coma, hypotension, respiratory depression, pulmonary edema, seizures	
Low level	N/A	
After event, time until…		
Negative result	2–3 days	May take up to 6 days with sustained-release formulations
Causes of spurious results	Rifampin, quinine, fluoroquinolones, poppy seeds	False positive
	Mefenamic acid	False negative
Additional info	N/A	

Partial Pressure of Arterial Carbon Dioxide (PaCO$_2$ or PCO$_2$)

PARAMETER	DESCRIPTION	COMMENTS
Common reference range	36–44 mm Hg	
Critical values	>70–80 mm Hg, consider mechanical ventilation	
Inherent activity	CO_2 serves as a volatile acid that can be exhaled	
Location	Measures partial pressure of CO_2 in arterial blood	
Causes of abnormal levels		
High	Opioids, benzodiazepines	Measured as part of ABG panel to evaluate acid/base status
	Inadequate ventilation, airway obstruction, pneumonia, pulmonary edema, impaired neuromuscular function at diaphragm	
Low	Salicylate intoxication, progesterone derivatives	
	Increased ventilation, pregnancy, high altitude, sepsis, hepatic failure	
Signs and symptoms		
High level	Respiratory failure	Acute changes of PaCO$_2$ are associated with greater drops of pH
Low level	Dizziness	
After event, time until…		
Initial elevation	Dependent on cause	
Peak values	Dependent on cause	
Normalization	Renal compensation: 3–5 days	
Causes of spurious results	Obtaining a venous sample	
Additional info	Not to be confused with venous total CO_2 or HCO_3 levels	

Partial Pressure of Arterial Oxygen (PaO$_2$ or PO$_2$)

PARAMETER	DESCRIPTION	COMMENTS
Common reference range	80–100 mm Hg	
Critical values	<60 mm Hg	
Inherent activity	Needed for cellular metabolism	
Location	Measures amount of O$_2$ in arterial blood	
Causes of abnormal levels		
High	Excess O$_2$ administration	Monitored if high FiO$_2$ gas administered or hypoxia suspected
Low	Hypoventilation, high altitude, ventilation/perfusion mismatch	
Signs and symptoms		
High level	Alveolar edema/hemorrhage, diminished lung compliance	
Low level	Hyperventilation (if disease process impairs gas exchange), cyanosis, mental status changes, seizures, coma	
After event, time until…	N/A	
Causes of spurious results	Venous sample, improper storage (not on ice with quick analysis), air bubbles in syringe	
Additional info	During PaO$_2$ values of 60–80 mm Hg, Hgb saturation is often 90% and O$_2$ may not be required	

PEFR (Peak Expiratory Flow Rate)

PARAMETER	DESCRIPTION	COMMENTS
Common reference range	>80% of best PEFR	
	Normals based on height, weight and gender	
Critical values	<50 % of personal best PEFR	
Inherent activity	N/A	Measured within first milliseconds of expiratory flow
Location	N/A	
Causes of abnormal levels		
High	N/A	
Low	Asthma exacerbation	
Signs and symptoms		
High level	N/A	
Low level	SOB, wheezing, coughing	
After event, time until…	N/A	
Causes of spurious results	Less useful in preschool patients and elderly	
Additional info	Used to determine severity of asthma exacerbation	

pH (of Arterial Blood)

PARAMETER	DESCRIPTION	COMMENTS
Common reference range	7.36–7.44	
Critical values	<7.2, >7.6	
Inherent activity	N/A	
Location	N/A	
Causes of abnormal levels		
High	Administration of basic pH medications (e.g., NaHCO$_3$)	Monitored if respiratory distress, desire to rule out acid/base conditions impacting patient's clinical status or with IV NaHCO$_3$ administration to correct acidosis
	Increased respiratory rate, decreased excretion of bicarbonate, emesis	
Low	Decreased respiratory rate/O$_2$ perfusion, increased excretion of bicarbonate (including diarrhea), administration of large volumes of pH neutral fluids (pH = 7), decreased circulation (e.g., shock)	
Signs and symptoms		
High level	Arteriolar constriction, hypoventilation (if metabolic in origin), hypokalemia, seizures, lethargy, stupor	Decreased respirations are compensatory
Low level	Increased respirations (if metabolic in origin), decreased cardiac output, hyperkalemia, altered mental status, coma	Increased respirations are compensatory
After event, time until…		
Initial elevation	Dependent on cause	Event: cause of pH disturbance
Peak values	Dependent on cause	
Normalization	Respiratory compensation: minutes to hours	
	Metabolic compensation: 3–5 days	
Causes of spurious results	Mixed acid-base disorders may result in a normal pH, inadvertent venous sample	
Additional info	Specimens must be transported to the lab quickly on ice	

Phencyclidine (PCP) (Urine Drug Screen)

PARAMETER	DESCRIPTION	COMMENTS
Common reference range	Negative	
Critical value	Positive	
Inherent activity	Yes	
Location		
Production	N/A	
Storage	N/A	
Secretion/excretion	N/A	
Causes of abnormal levels		
High	Ingestion, smoking, snorting, injection of PCP	
Low	N/A	
Signs and symptoms		
High level	Hallucinations, schizophrenia-like behavior, hypertension, hyperthermia, diaphoresis, tachycardia, nystagmus, ataxia, depressed respirations, seizures, coma	Related to higher doses
Low level	N/A	
After event, time until…		
Negative result from sporadic use	2–10 days	
Negative result from chronic use	Weeks or months	May persist for longer period of time with heavy, long-term use or massive overdose preceded by chronic use
Causes of spurious results	Dextromethorphan, ketamine, diphenhydramine, sertraline	False-positive result
Additional info	N/A	

Phenobarbital/Primidone

PARAMETER	DESCRIPTION	COMMENTS
Common reference range	Phenobarbital: 15–40 mg/L	Level can be drawn any time during interval (long half-life)
	Primidone: 5–12 mg/L	Concentrations up to 70 mg/L may be needed for status epilepticus
Critical values	>40 mg/L	
Inherent activity	Anticonvulsant activity at GABA receptors	
Location	N/A	
Causes of abnormal levels		
High	Phenobarbital, primidone	
	Medications that inhibit 2C9 and 2C19	
	Valproic acid can increase levels	
Low	Medications that induce 2C9 and 2C19	
Signs and symptoms		
High level	Sedation, ataxia, stupor, coma, hypotension, bradycardia	
Low level	N/A	
After event, time until…		
Normalization	Steady state may require up to 3 wk	
Causes of spurious results	N/A	
Additional info	Phenobarbital is a metabolite of primidone	

Phenytoin

PARAMETER	DESCRIPTION	COMMENTS
Common reference range	Adult: 10–20 mg/L	Trough level recommended
	Infant: 6–11 mg/L	
	Unbound: 1–2 mg/L	Check level at least 4 hr after fosphenytoin administration
		Unbound range depends on temperature of sample
Critical values	>30 mg/L associated with ADRs	
Inherent activity	Alters sodium transport across membranes resulting in anticonvulsant activity	
Location	N/A	
Causes of abnormal levels		
High	Phenytoin/fosphenytoin	
Low	Antacids may decrease absorption, folic acid may increase metabolism, valproic acid, salicylates, NSAIDs displace phenytoin	
	Diseases and drugs causing decreased protein binding may cause falsely low total levels	
Signs and symptoms		
High level	Nystagmus, CNS depression (ataxia, confusion, drowsiness), coma, seizures, hypotension if administered at >50 mg/min IV	
Low level	N/A	
After event, time until…		
Normalization	Up to 3 wk for steady-state	
Causes of spurious results	Protein binding interactions, doxycycline, metronidazole, ibuprofen, theophylline	
Additional info	Corrected level = measured/$[(N \times albumin) + 0.1]$	
	X = 0.2 if low albumin and CrCl >25 mL/min	
	X = 0.1 if renal failure	
	Fosphenytoin is an IV prodrug of phenytoin	

Phosphate

PARAMETER	DESCRIPTION	COMMENTS
Common reference range		
Adults	2.6–4.5 mg/dL (0.84–1.45 mmol/L)	
Newborn (0–5 days old)	4.8–8.2 mg/dL (1.55–2.65 mmol/L)	
Pediatrics (1–3 yr old)	3.8–6.5 mg/dL (1.25–2.1 mmol/L)	
Pediatrics (4–11 yr old)	3.7–5.6 mg/dL (1.2–1.8 mmol/L)	
Pediatrics (12–15 yr old)	2.9–5.4 mg/dL (0.95–1.75 mmol/L)	
Children (16–19 yr old)	2.7–4.7 mg/dL (0.9–1.5 mmol/L)	
Critical value	>8 or <1 mg/dL (>2.6 or <0.3 mmol/L)	Acute changes more dangerous than chronic abnormalities
Inherent activity	Yes	Bone and tooth integrity, phospholipid synthesis, acid-base balance, calcium homeostasis, enzyme activation, formation of high-energy bonds
Location		
Storage	ECF, cell membrane structure, ICF, collagen, bone	85% in bone
Secretion/ excretion	Filtration by kidneys	Mostly reabsorbed
Causes of abnormal levels		
High	Vitamin D, phosphate-based medications	
	Renal failure, extracellular shifting, increased intake of dietary phosphate or vitamin D	
Low	Phosphate binders (Ca, Mg, Al-based, sevelamer, lanthanum)	Listed drugs are commonly monitored
	Increased renal excretion, intracellular shifting (e.g., with refeeding syndrome), decreased intake of phosphate or vitamin D	
Signs and symptoms		
High level	Neuromuscular (fatigue, depression, memory loss, hallucinations, seizures, tetany), QT prolongation	Due primarily to hypocalcemia and hyperparathyroidism
Low level	Bone pain, weakness, malaise, hypocalcemia, cardiac failure, respiratory failure	Usually due to diminished intracellular ATP and erythrocyte 2,3-DPG concentrations

(continued)

Phosphate (Cont.)

After event, time until...

Initial elevation	Usually over months to years
Peak values	Usually over months to years
Normalization	Over days with renal transplantation
Causes of spurious results	Hemolyzed samples (falsely elevated) and methotrexate (falsely elevated)
Additional info	N/A

Plasma Glucose

PARAMETER	DESCRIPTION	COMMENTS
Common reference range		
Adults and Children	Fasting: 70–110 mg/dL 2 hr postprandial: <140 mg/dL	ADA advises that fasting levels >100 increase risk for diabetes and >125 are consistent with diabetes; they advocate a fasting goal of 70–130 and postprandial goal of <180 for nonpregnant adults with diabetes
Pregnant	Fasting <92, 1 hr post OGTT <180, 2 hr post OGTT <153 mg/dL	
Full-term infant	20–90 mg/dL	
Critical value	No previous history: >200 mg/dL	
	Anytime: <50 mg/dL	
Inherent activity	Yes	Major source of energy for cellular metabolism
Location		
Production	Liver and muscle	Dietary intake
Storage	Liver and muscle	As glycogen
Secretion/excretion	Mostly metabolized for energy	Levels >180 mg/dL spill into urine
Causes of abnormal levels		
High	Steroids, thiazides, epinephrine, glucagon	Glucose commonly monitored when taking systemic steroids
	Diabetes mellitus type I & II, excess carbohydrate intake, stress (physiologic)	
Low	Insulin secretion/dose excessive relative to diet, hypoglycemic agents, insulinomas, impaired renal function (and receiving insulin)	Most common in diabetics as a result of therapy/nutrition imbalances
Signs and symptoms		
High level	Polyuria, polydipsia, polyphagia, weakness	Long-term: damage to kidneys, retina, neurons, and blood vessels
Low level	Hunger, sweating, weakness, trembling, headache, confusion, seizures, coma	From neuroglycopenia and adrenergic discharge
After event, time until...		
Initial elevation	After steroids: hours	
	After epinephrine or glucagon: minutes	
Normalization	After insulin: minutes (depends on insulin type)	
Causes of spurious results	Metronidazole high dose, vitamin C (falsely low)	With some automated assays
Additional info	Many glucometers use an adjustment factor to estimate plasma blood glucose	

Platelet Count

PARAMETER	DESCRIPTION	COMMENTS
Common reference range		
Adults	140,000–440,000/μL	
Newborns	84,000–478,000/μL	
Children (1–10 yr old)	150,000–600,000/μL	
Critical value	>800,000 or <20,000/μL	
Inherent activity	Yes	
Location		
Production	Bone marrow	Also can be produced by lungs and other tissues
Storage	Not stored	⅔ found in circulation, ⅓ found in spleen
Secretion/ excretion	Destroyed by spleen, liver, bone marrow	
Causes of abnormal levels		
High	Stress, infection, splenectomy, RA, chronic pancreatitis	
Low	Heparins, PCNs/CSNs, sulfonamides, linezolid, vancomycin, antineoplastics, valproic acid, GP2b3a antagonists, quinidine	Heparins, antineoplastics, valproic acid, GP2b3a antagonists commonly monitored
	Hemorrhage, TTP, ITP, aplastic anemia, leukemia, splenomegaly	Linezolid monitored with prolonged use (>2 wk)
Signs and symptoms		
High level	Thrombosis: CVA, DVT, PE, portal vein thrombosis	
Low level	Bleeding: mucosal, cutaneous	CNS bleeding (i.e., intracranial hemorrhage) is most common cause of death in patients with thrombocytopenia
After event, time until…		
Initial elevation	Days to weeks	
Peak values	Days to weeks	
Normalization	Weeks to months	
Causes of spurious results	Values outside 50,000–500,000/μL, Hct <20 or >50%	Need to perform manual counts in these instances
Additional info	Average platelet lifespan is 8–12 days	

Polymorphonuclear Neutrophils

PARAMETER	DESCRIPTION	COMMENTS
Common reference range	45% to 73%	
Critical value	<500 cells/mm³	
Inherent activity	Yes	Exists to ingest and digest foreign proteins (e.g., bacteria and fungi)
Location		
Production	Bone marrow	
Storage	Bone marrow, vascular endothelium	
Secretion/ excretion	N/A	
Causes of abnormal levels		
High	Corticosteroids, epinephrine, lithium, G-CSF, GM-CSF	G-CSF and GM-CSF commonly monitored
	Acute/chronic bacterial infection, trauma, MI, leukemia	
Low	Antineoplastic cytotoxic agents, captopril, cephalosporins, chloramphenicol, clozapine, ganciclovir, methimazole, penicillins, phenothiazines, procainamide, ticlopidine, tricyclic antidepressants, vancomycin	Antineoplastic/cytotoxic agents, chloramphenicol, clozapine, ganciclovir, methimazole, ticlopidine commonly monitored
	Radiation exposure, vitamin B12 or folate deficiency, salmonellosis, pertussis, overwhelming bacterial infection	
Signs and symptoms		
High level	Related to underlying cause	
Low level	Related to underlying cause	
After event, time until…		
Initial elevation	N/A	
Peak values	N/A	
Normalization	N/A	
Causes of spurious results	N/A	
Additional info	N/A	

Potassium

PARAMETER	DESCRIPTION	COMMENTS
Common reference range		
Adults	3.5–5.0 mEq/L (3.5–5.0 mmol/L)	
Premature neonates (48 hr of life)	3.0–6.0 mEq/L (3.0–6.0 mmol/L)	
Newborns	3.7–5.9 mEq/L (3.7–5.9 mmol/L)	
Infants	4.1–5.3 mEq/L (4.1–5.3 mmol/L)	
Children	3.4–4.7 mEq/L (3.4–4.7 mmol/L)	
Critical value	>7 or <2.5 mEq/L (>7 or <2.5 mmol/L)	Acute changes more dangerous than chronic abnormalities
Inherent activity	Yes	Control of muscle and nervous tissue excitability, acid–base balance, intracellular fluid balance
Location		
Storage	98% in intracellular fluid	
Secretion/excretion	Mostly secreted by distal nephron	Some via GI tract secretion
Causes of abnormal levels		
High	ACEIs, ARAs, ARBs, amphotericin B, triamterene, beta blockers, trimethoprim, heparin	Commonly monitored with ACEIs, ARAs, ARBs, amphotericin B, triamterene, trimethoprim
	Renal failure (GFR <10 mL/min), acidosis, rhabdomyolysis, Addison's disease	
Low	Insulin, beta agonists, diuretics (loop/TZD), corticosteroids	Commonly monitored with insulin (especially at high doses or on infusion), beta agonists (occasionally), diuretics (loop/TZD)
	CHF, cirrhosis, nephrotic syndrome, alkalosis, vomiting, diarrhea, malabsorption, alcoholism, hyperaldosteronism	
Signs and symptoms		
High level	ECG changes, bradycardia, hypotension, cardiac arrest	
Low level	ECG changes, arrhythmias, hyperreflexia, cramps, ileus, urinary retention	
After event, time until...		
Initial elevation	Variable	The faster the change, the more dangerous the consequences
Peak values	Variable	
Normalization	Days, if renal function is normal	Faster with appropriate treatment
Causes of spurious results	Hemolyzed samples (falsely elevated)	High potassium content in erythrocytes
Additional info	Low vitamin K can potentiate digoxin toxicity	

Prealbumin

PARAMETER	DESCRIPTION	COMMENTS
Common reference range	19.5–35.8 mg/dL	
Critical value	N/A	
Inherent activity	Yes	Carrier protein
Location		
Production	Liver	
Storage	Serum	
Secretion/ excretion	Kidney	
Causes of abnormal levels		
High	N/A	
Low	Malnutrition, infection	Negative acute phase reactant
Signs and symptoms		
High level	N/A	
Low level	Signs and symptoms of poor nutrition	
After event, time until…		
Initial depression	Days	
Lowest values	Days to weeks	Half-life about 2–3 days
Normalization	Days	
Causes of spurious results	N/A	
Additional info	More sensitive to protein nutrition than albumin	
	Less affected by liver disease than albumin	

Procainamide

PARAMETER	DESCRIPTION	COMMENTS
Common reference range	4–8 mg/L	Trough level recommended (within 1 hr of next dose)
	Up to 12 mg/L needed for some	
	NAPA: 5–30 mg/L	
Critical values	>12 mg/L	
Inherent activity	Antiarrhythmic	
Location	N/A	
Causes of abnormal levels		
High	Cimetidine and trimethoprim compete for excretion, 2D6 inhibitors (e.g., amiodarone), fluoroquinolones, and quinidine	Commonly monitored if prolonged infusions or renal/hepatic impairment
	Renal/heart failure	
	NAPA levels increase with renal impairment	
Low	Ethanol	
Signs and symptoms		
High level	>8 mg/L: anorexia, N/V/D, weakness, hypotension	
	>12 mg/L: heart block, ventricular arrhythmias, cardiac arrest, TdP	
Low level	N/A	
After event, time until...		
Normalization	Up to 18 hr until steady state	
Causes of spurious results	N/A	
Additional info	NAPA metabolite has type III antiarrhythmic properties	

Progesterone

PARAMETER	DESCRIPTION	COMMENTS
Common reference range		
Adult women, early in cycle	37–57 ng/dL	
Adult women, midcycle	Rising	
Adult women, luteal phase	332–1198 ng/dL	
Menopausal women	10–22 ng/dL	
Critical values	N/A	Extremely high or low values should be reported quickly
Inherent activity	Yes	Facilitates implantation of fertilized oocyte
Location	Produced by corpus luteum	
Causes of abnormal levels		
High	Valproic acid, clomiphene, corticotropin, ketoconazole, progesterone, tamoxifen	Commonly monitored with clomiphene, progesterone
	Congenital adrenal hyperplasia, ovarian tumor	
Low	Ampicillin, carbamazepine, phenytoin, danazol, GnRH agonists, oral contraceptives, pravastatin	
	Spontaneous abortion	
Signs and symptoms		
High level	↑17-OHP, ↑DHEAS, ↓cortisol, hirsutism/acne, virilization, rapid progression of symptoms	Dependent on cause
Low level	Vaginal bleeding	
After event, time until…	N/A	
Causes of spurious results	N/A	
Additional info	Infertility commonly monitored with test; midluteal progesterone <6 ng/mL suggests ovulation	

Prolactin

PARAMETER	DESCRIPTION	COMMENTS
Common reference range		
Children	1–20 ng/mL	Obtain 12-hr fasting samples in the morning
Adult women	1–25 ng/mL	
Menopausal women	1–20 ng/mL	
Critical values	Levels >100 ng/mL in nonlactating females may indicate a prolactin-secreting tumor	Extremely high or low values should be reported quickly
Inherent activity	Yes	Initiates and maintains lactation
Location	Anterior pituitary	Release of prolactin is inhibited by dopamine secreted by hypothalamus
Causes of abnormal levels		
High	Dopamine antagonists (e.g., antipsychotics, methyldopa), antihistamines, estrogen, GnRH, insulin, megestrol, metoclopramide, MAOIs, opiates, phenytoin, verapamil	Monitor if symptoms suggest excess prolactin
	Pituitary adenoma, hypothyroidism (primary), PCOS, anorexia nervosa	
Low	Dopaminergic agonists (e.g., bromocriptine, L-dopa), clonidine, carbamazepine, dexamethasone, nifedipine, tamoxifen	
Signs and symptoms		
High level	Galactorrhea/visual changes, coarse skin and hair, hirsutism/acne/obesity, cachexia/low BMI	Depends on cause
Low level	N/A	
After event, time until…	N/A	
Causes of spurious results	Increased values are associated with newborns, pregnancy, postpartum period, stress, exercise, sleep, nipple stimulation and lactation	
Additional info	Pituitary adenoma monitored with this test	Can assess effectiveness of surgery, chemotherapy, or radiation for prolactin secreting tumors

Protein C & S

PARAMETER	DESCRIPTION	COMMENTS
Common reference range	Protein C: 70% to 140% Protein S: 70% to 140%	Protein C and S levels lower in childhood/infancy and are assay dependent; protein S levels lower in women
Critical values	N/A	
Inherent activity	Activated protein C is an anticoagulant Protein S has anticoagulant properties and facilitates protein C activity	
Location		
Produced	Liver	
Causes of abnormal levels		
High	N/A	
Low	Protein C: genetic deficiency/sepsis Protein S: genetic deficiency/estrogen/ pregnancy	
Signs and symptoms		
High level	N/A	
Low level	Thrombosis (venous), purple toe	
After event, time until…	N/A	
Causes of spurious results	Anticoagulant use cause low levels due to inhibition (but this might not be the cause of thrombosis); elevated factor VIII can cause falsely low protein S functional assays; lupus anticoagulant can increase values of protein S	Generally advised to wait 2 wk after anticoagulation to test
Additional info	Levels not recommended until at least 10 days after VTE identified	

PSA (Prostate-Specific Antigen)

PARAMETER	DESCRIPTION	COMMENTS
Common reference range	<4 ng/mL	Some experts recommend using age-dependent ranges instead
Critical values	≥10 ng/mL is highly suggestive of prostate cancer	Extremely high values should be reported quickly
Inherent activity	Yes	Responsible for liquefying semen after ejaculation
Location	Produced in transition zone of prostate gland	
Causes of abnormal levels		
High	Exogenous testosterone supplements	PSA monitored with testosterone supplements
	Prostate cancer, BPH, prostatitis, prostate trauma, prostate surgery, acute urinary retention, ejaculation, exercise, bicycling	
Low	N/A	
Signs and symptoms		
High level	Asymptomatic, voiding symptoms, metastatic symptoms (e.g., bone pain)	
Low level	N/A	
After event, time until…		
Initial elevation	After prostate manipulation, the PSA levels will increase within hours	
Peak values	N/A	
Normalization	Prostate massage: days	
	Transurethral prostatectomy: weeks	
	Effective treatment of prostate cancer: days to weeks	
Causes of spurious results	N/A	
Additional info	Used to monitor prostate cancer	

Quinidine

PARAMETER	DESCRIPTION	COMMENTS
Common reference range	2–5 mg/L	Trough level recommended (within 1 hr of next dose)
Critical values	>6 mg/L	
Inherent activity	Antiarrhythmic/antimalarial	
Location	N/A	
Causes of abnormal levels		
High	3A4 inhibitors, PGP inhibitors, many other drugs	
Low	3A4 inducers (including phenytoin)	
Signs and symptoms		
High level	Anorexia, nausea, diarrhea, cinchonism (blurred vision, lightheadedness, tremor, giddiness, and tinnitus), hypotension, ventricular arrhythmias	
Low level	N/A	
After event, time until…		
Normalization	Up to 3 days until steady state	
Causes of spurious results	Quinine can interfere with immunoassay	
	Disease states (including MI) causing elevated levels of alpha-1-acid glycoprotein may require higher levels to exert desired effect	
Additional info	N/A	

RBC Distribution Width (RDW)

PARAMETER	DESCRIPTION	COMMENTS
Common reference range	11.5% to 14.5%	
Critical values	N/A	
Inherent activity	N/A	Estimates variability in RBC size
Location	N/A	
Causes of abnormal levels		
High	Mixed anemias (micro and macrocytic), iron deficiency anemia, B12/folate deficiency	Monitored to help identify cause of anemia
Low	Normal levels in hemolytic anemia, acute blood loss	
Signs and symptoms		
High level	Dependent on type of anemia	
Low level	Dependent on type of anemia	
After event, time until…	N/A	
Causes of spurious results	N/A	
Additional info	RDW = standard deviation of MCV/ mean value of MCV	

Red Blood Cells (RBC)

PARAMETER	DESCRIPTION	COMMENTS
Common reference range		
Adults	Males: $4.5–5.9 \times 10^6$ cells/μL	
	Females: $4.1–5.1 \times 10^6$ cells/μL	
Newborns (1–3 days old)	5.3×10^6 cells/μL	
1 wk old	5.1×10^6 cells/μL	
2 wk old	4.9×10^6 cells/μL	
1 mo old	4.2×10^6 cells/μL	
2 mo old	3.8×10^6 cells/μL	
3–6 mo old	3.8×10^6 cells/μL	
0.5–2 yr old	4.5×10^6 cells/μL	
2–6 yr old	4.6×10^6 cells/μL	
6–12 yr old	4.6×10^6 cells/μL	
12–18 yr old	Males: 4.9×10^6 cells/μL	
	Females: 4.6×10^6 cells/μL	
18–49 yr old	Males: 5.2×10^6 cells/μL	
	Females: 4.6×10^6 cells/μL	
Critical values	N/A	
Inherent activity	Deliver O_2 to tissues and exchange for CO_2	
Location	Circulatory system	
Causes of abnormal levels		
High	Androgens, ESAs	
	Polycythemia (e.g., as a result from hypoxia), renal artery stenosis, high altitude	
Low	Under-production (e.g., due to deficiency of factors involved like iron, folate or vit B_{12}), loss of blood (can occur occultly), premature RBC destruction (e.g., hemolytic anemia)	Hgb/Hct more commonly used to diagnose anemia
Signs and symptoms		
High level	Dependent on cause	
Low level	Fatigue, pallor, bleeding	
After event, time until...		
Normalization	Commonly takes 6–8 wk to return levels to normal (depending on disease process)	Event: anemia
Causes of spurious results	N/A	
Additional info	Erythrocytes have a lifespan of 120 days	

Reticulocyte Count

PARAMETER	DESCRIPTION	COMMENTS
Common reference range	0.5% to 2.5% of RBCs	
Critical values	N/A	
Inherent activity	N/A	Immature form of RBC
Location	Bone marrow, blood	
Causes of abnormal levels		
High	Acute blood loss, hemolysis	Monitored to help identify cause of anemia
Low	Bone marrow suppression	
Signs and symptoms		
High level	Pallor, fatigue, evidence of bleed, jaundice	
Low level	Dependent on cause (and the blood lines that are suppressed)	
After event, time until...		
Initial elevation	Reticulocytes can increase after 5–7 days after starting iron or vitamins that were deficient	Event: replaced deficiency of iron/vitamins
Causes of spurious results	Low Hct	
Additional info	Reticulocyte index = % reticulocytes × (actual Hct/normal Hct)	
	Commonly ordered to help distinguish hypoproliferative disorders from those causing acute loss of RBCs	

Rheumatoid Factor

PARAMETER	DESCRIPTION	COMMENTS
Common reference range	Negative	
Critical value	Concentration: >20 International Units/mL	
	Titer: >1:20	
Inherent activity	Yes	Immunoglobulins that are directed against the Fc portion of IgG
Location		
Production	N/A	
Storage	Blood	
Secretion/excretion	N/A	
Causes of abnormal levels		
High	Rheumatoid arthritis, SLE, systemic sclerosis, mixed connective-tissue disease, Sjögren's syndrome	
	Mononucleosis, hepatitis, malaria, tuberculosis, syphilis, subacute bacterial endocarditis, chronic liver disease	Nonrheumatic diseases
Low	N/A	
Signs and symptoms		
High level	Related to underlying cause	
Low level	N/A	
After event, time until…		
Initial elevation	N/A	
Peak values	N/A	
Normalization	N/A	
Causes of spurious results	N/A	
Additional info	While elevated levels are common in RA, rheumatoid factor is neither very sensitive nor specific for RA; it should be used in context of patient presentation	

Salicylate

PARAMETER	DESCRIPTION	COMMENTS
Common reference range	Anti-inflammatory: 100–250 mg/L	Trough recommended
	Analgesic/antipyretic: 20–100 mg/L	
Critical values	N/A	
Inherent activity	Inhibition of prostaglandin synthesis	
Location	N/A	
Causes of abnormal levels		
High	Aspirin (if overdose suspected), salicylate-based medications	Monitored if suspected overdose
	Pregnancy, liver disease, nephrotic syndrome, uremia all increase unbound fractions	
Low	Nonadherence	
Signs and symptoms		
High level	Tinnitus, bleeding, N/V, hyperventilation, metabolic acidosis, renal failure	
Low level	N/A	
After event, time until…		
Normalization	Steady state at 1 wk	
Causes of spurious results	Low protein states can cause a falsely low level	Therapeutic range for unbound salicylate does not exist
	Diflunisal can cause false positives	
Additional info	Toxicity can occur at levels within reference range	

Serotonin Release Assay (SRA)

PARAMETER	DESCRIPTION	COMMENTS
Common reference range	Negative	Sensitive and specific but costly and time consuming
Critical values	Positive	
Inherent activity	N/A	
Location	N/A	
Causes of abnormal levels		
High	Heparin exposure (more common with UFH than LMWH)	Not routinely monitored w/UFH/LMWH unless HIT suspected
Low	N/A	
Signs and symptoms		
High level	Thrombosis (venous and arterial), skin lesions, chills/cardiorespiratory distress after UFH bolus	
Low level	N/A	
After event, time until…	N/A	
Causes of spurious results	N/A	
Additional info	Commonly ordered after a positive ELISA test to confirm diagnosis of HIT	Commonly, platelets decrease 5–14 days after heparin but can decrease in 1 day if previous exposure

Serum Creatinine (SCr)

PARAMETER	DESCRIPTION	COMMENTS
Common reference range		
Adults	0.7–1.5 mg/dL	
Newborns	0.3–1.0 mg/dL	
Infants	0.2–0.4 mg/dL	
Children	0.3–0.7 mg/dL	
Adolescents	0.5–1.0 mg/dL	
Critical value	>⅓ elevation from baseline	
Inherent activity	No	
Location		
Production	Muscle	Spontaneous breakdown product of creatine and creatine phosphate
Storage	Serum	
Secretion/excretion	Kidney	
Causes of abnormal levels		
High	Trimethoprim, cimetidine, flucytosine, ACE-I/ARB, NSAIDs, aminoglycosides, cyclosporine, amphotericin, contrast dye	Listed medications (with exception of cimetidine) are commonly monitored
	Recent meat ingestion	
	Renal failure, rhabdomyolysis	
Low	Decreased hepatic synthesis of creatine	Precursor of creatinine
	Decreased muscle mass (e.g., elderly)	Amputation, malnutrition, muscle wasting
Signs and symptoms		
High level	N/A	
Low level	Related to underlying disorder	
After event, time until…		
Initial elevation	N/A	
Peak values	N/A	
Normalization	N/A	
Causes of spurious results	Uric acid, glucose, fructose, acetone, pyruvic acid, ascorbic acid	Large amounts in the serum can lead to falsely elevated levels
	Elevated bilirubin	Falsely low SCr
Additional info	In otherwise healthy stable patients, the rate of creatinine production equals excretion	
	Standardization of SCr with isotope dilution mass spectrometry has reduced interlaboratory variation of SCr values and reduced SCr by 5% to 20% compared with pre-standardization values	

Serum Osmolality

PARAMETER	DESCRIPTION	COMMENTS
Common reference range	280–300 mOsm/L	
Critical values	>325 mOsm/L, <265 mOsm/L	
Inherent activity	Measures solute concentration	
Location	Serum	
Causes of abnormal levels		
High	Alcohols, hypernatremia, uremia, hyperglycemia	
Low	Hyponatremia, ADH release	
Signs and symptoms		
High level	Neurologic changes	
Low level	Dependent on cause	
After event, time until…	N/A	
Causes of spurious results	Alcohols (including methanol and ethylene glycol) cause a discrepancy between calculated osmolality and measured	
Additional info	Osmolal gap = measured – calculated osmolality (considered positive if >10)	Calculated osmolality = (Na × 2) + (glucose (mg/dL)/18) + (BUN (mg/dL)/2.8)

Sirolimus

PARAMETER	DESCRIPTION	COMMENTS
Common reference range	When used with cyclosporine and corticosteroids: 5–15 mcg/L	Whole blood samples preferred
	When used with MMF and corticosteroids: 8–12 mcg/L	Trough levels recommended
		Ranges depend on concurrent immunosuppressants
Critical values	N/A	
Inherent activity	Immunosuppressant	
Location	N/A	
Causes of abnormal levels		
High	3A4 and P-gp inhibitors	Drug levels commonly monitored for safety/efficacy
Low	3A4 inducers	
Signs and symptoms		
High level	Nephrotoxicity, dyslipidemia, thrombocytopenia	
Low level	Organ rejection	
After event, time until…	At least 6 days until steady state	
Causes of spurious results	N/A	
Additional info	Chromatographic methods preferred to measure levels	

Sodium

PARAMETER	DESCRIPTION	COMMENTS
Common reference range		
Adults	136–145 mEq/L	
Pediatrics: premature infants (48 hr of life)	128–148 mEq/L	
Pediatrics: newborns	133–146 mEq/L	
Pediatrics: infants	139–146 mEq/L	
Pediatrics: children	138–145 mEq/L	
Critical value	>160 or <120 mEq/L	Acute changes more dangerous than chronic abnormalities
Inherent activity	Yes	Maintenance of transmembrane electric potential
Location		
Storage	Mostly in ECF	
Secretion/excretion	Filtered by kidneys, mostly reabsorbed; some secretion in distal nephron	Closely related to water homeostasis
Causes of abnormal levels		
High	Lithium, demeclocycline, foscarnet, hypertonic saline administration	Listed drugs are commonly monitored (hypertonic saline monitored several times daily)
	Diabetes insipidus, inability to express thirst	
Low	TZD diuretics, carbamazepine, cyclophosphamide, NSAIDs, SSRIs, TCAs, phenothiazines, ecstasy, hypotonic fluids	Diuretics, carbamazepine, hypotonic fluids commonly monitored
	Hypervolemic: CHF, cirrhosis, nephrosis	
	Euvolemic: SIADH, head trauma/bleed/mass, lung cancer, hypothyroidism	
	Hypovolemic: diarrhea, adrenal insufficiency	
Signs and symptoms		
High level	Lethargy, muscle twitching, seizures, restlessness, coma, death	Overly rapid elevation of serum Na can cause contraction of CSF volume, resulting in neurological sequelae
Low level	Disorientation, lethargy, muscle cramps, nausea, seizures, hypothermia, depressed reflexes, agitation	Overly rapid depression of serum Na can cause expansion of CSF volume, resulting in neurological sequelae

(continued)

Sodium (Cont.)

After event, time until...		
Initial elevation	Variable	The faster the change, the more dangerous the consequences
Peak values	Variable	
Normalization	Days, if renal function is normal	Faster with appropriate treatment
Causes of spurious results	Hyperglycemia can cause pseudohyponatremia	
Additional info	For every 100 mg/dL increase in blood glucose, serum Na decreases by 1.7 mEq/L	

Tacrolimus (FK506)

PARAMETER	DESCRIPTION	COMMENTS
Common reference range	**Kidney transplant** with MMF/IL-2 receptor antagonist mo 1–12: 4–11 mcg/L	Whole blood sample preferred Generally, trough recommended (at least 12 hr postdose)
	Liver transplant mo 1–12: 5–20 mcg/L	
	Heart transplant mo 1–3: 10–20 mcg/L mo >3: 5–15 mcg/L after 12 mo: 5–10 mcg/L	
Critical values	>20 mcg/L	
Inherent activity	Immunosuppressant	
Location	N/A	
Causes of abnormal levels		
High	Renal impairment, 3A4 inhibitors	Drug levels commonly monitored for safety/efficacy
Low	3A4 inducers	
Signs and symptoms		
High level	Nephrotoxicity, neurotoxicity	
Low level	Organ rejection	
After event, time until...		
Normalization	Up to 5 days to reach steady state	
Causes of spurious results	Elevated hematocrit can cause falsely low readings with microparticle enzyme immunoassay	
Additional info	HPLC method preferred if patient has liver disease	

Testosterone

PARAMETER	DESCRIPTION	COMMENTS
Common reference range		
Children	0.12–0.16 ng/dL	Unbound (free) is active form and has different reference ranges
Adult males	280–1100 ng/dL	
Adult women	0.25–0.67 ng/dL	Draw levels between 6–10 a.m.
Menopausal women	0.21–0.37 ng/dL	
Critical values	>200 ng/dL in females indicates virilizing tumor	<200 ng/dL in males associated with symptomatic hypogonadism
Inherent activity	Yes	Males: secondary sex characteristics, sexual drive, bone mass, prostate enlargement, spermatogenesis
Location	Men: produced in testes	
	Women: adrenal glands and ovaries	
Causes of abnormal levels		
High	Danazol, phenytoin, rifampin, clomiphene, dopamine agonists, gonadotropin, tamoxifen	Monitored if administering exogenous testosterone
	Adrenal neoplasms, congenital adrenal hyperplasia, ovarian tumors, PCOS, Cushing's syndrome, hyperthyroidism, excessive exercise	
Low	Alcohol, carbamazepine, androgens, cimetidine, dexamethasone, diethylstilbestrol, digoxin, estrogen, ketoconazole, GnRH agonists, medroxyprogesterone, phenothiazines, spironolactone, tetracycline	Monitor if symptoms suggest low levels
	Males: hypogonadism, hypopituitarism, orchiectomy, cirrhosis, age >50, hyperprolactinemia, hypothyroidism	
Signs and symptoms		
High level	Virilization, ↑DHEAS, ↑or ↓cortisol, ↑17-OHP, hirsutism/acne/obesity, buffalo hump/obesity/striae, mood swings, increased libido	Depends on cause
Low level	Males: decreased libido, erectile dysfunction, gynecomastia, weight gain	

(continued)

Testosterone (Cont.)

After event, time until…	N/A	
Causes of spurious results	N/A	
Additional info	Used to detect ovarian tumors and virilizing conditions in women and evaluate hypogonadism in males	Conditions that significantly alter the concentration of SHBG can increase or decrease the concentration of free testosterone

Theophylline

PARAMETER	DESCRIPTION	COMMENTS
Common reference range	Adult: 5–15 mg/L	Trough level recommended
	Neonates: 5–13 mg/L	Levels up to 20 mg/L may be needed for effect in some
Critical values	>30 mg/L associated with dangerous ADEs	
Inherent activity	Bronchodilation, CNS stimulation, cardiovascular stimulation	
Location	N/A	
Causes of abnormal levels		
High	Theophylline, aminophylline	Levels routinely monitored with listed medications
	Liver disease, heart failure, drugs that inhibit 3A4 or 1A2	
Low	Smoking increases clearance, drugs that induce 3A4 or 1A2	
Signs and symptoms		
High level	>15 mg/L: N/V/D, irritability, insomnia	Higher: seizures, brain damage, death
	>40 mg/L: supraventricular tachycardia, hypotension, ventricular arrhythmias	
Low level	N/A	
After event, time until…		
Normalization	Steady state in 24 hr in nonsmokers (variable)	
Causes of spurious results	Caffeine, theobromine, APAP, doxycycline, levodopa, rifampin	
Additional info	Toxicity possible in the reference range	

Thiopurine Methyltransferase (TPMT)

PARAMETER	DESCRIPTION	COMMENTS
Common reference range	5–12 units/mL	Enzymatic testing of red blood cell lysate
Critical value	<5 units/mL	
	>12 units/mL	
Inherent activity	Yes	Enzyme responsible for the conversion of azathioprine and 6-mercaptopurine into inactive metabolites
Location		
Production	N/A	
Storage	Serum	
Secretion/excretion	N/A	
Causes of abnormal levels		
High	Gene mutation	
Low	Salicylate	
	Gene mutation	
Signs and symptoms		
High level	N/A	
Low level	Bone marrow toxicity	Related to elevated levels of azathioprine and 6-mercaptopurine
	Liver toxicity	
After event, time until…		
Initial elevation	N/A	
Peak values	N/A	
Normalization	N/A	
Causes of spurious results	N/A	
Additional info	FDA recommends that TPMT testing be done prior to initiation of 6-mercaptopurine	

Thyroid Stimulating Hormone (TSH)

PARAMETER	DESCRIPTION	COMMENTS
Common reference range	0.25–6.7 milliunits/L	Extremely high or low values should be reported quickly
Critical value	N/A	
Inherent activity	Yes	Stimulates thyroid to secrete hormones
Location		
Production	Anterior pituitary	
Storage	Anterior pituitary	
Secretion/excretion	Unknown	
Causes of abnormal levels		
High	Antithyroid drugs (e.g., methimazole/PTU), amiodarone, dopamine antagonists	Levels commonly monitored with antithyroid drugs and amiodarone
	Hypothyroidism	
Low	T4/T3 supplements, amiodarone, dopamine agonists, glucocorticoids	Levels commonly monitored with T4/T3 supplements and amiodarone
	Hyperthyroidism	
Signs and symptoms		
High level	Lethargy, constipation, dry skin, cold intolerance, slow speech, confusion	
Low level	Nervousness, weight loss, heat intolerance, HR increase, diaphoresis	
After event, time until…		
Initial elevation	Weeks to months	
Peak values	Weeks to months	
Normalization	Normally same time as onset	
Causes of spurious results	Pregnancy can cause falsely elevated readings	
Additional info	N/A	

Total Bilirubin

PARAMETER	DESCRIPTION	COMMENTS
Common reference range		
Adults	0.3–1.0 mg/dL	Varies with assay
Full-term neonates (0–1 day old)	<8.7 mg/dL	
Full-term neonates (1–2 days old)	<11.5 mg/dL	
Full-term neonates (3–5 days old)	<12 mg/dL	
Full-term neonates (>5 days old)	<1.2 mg/dL	
Critical value (adults)	>4 mg/dL	In adults
Inherent activity	Yes	CNS irritant or toxin in high levels in newborn (not adult)
Location		
Production	Liver	
Storage	Gallbladder	
Secretion/excretion	Stool and urine	Excreted into bile; bilirubin and urobilinogen
Causes of abnormal levels		
High	Liver disease (both hepatocellular and cholestatic), hemolysis, metabolic abnormalities	
Low	N/A	
Signs and symptoms		
High level	Jaundice, pruritus, dark urine, clay-colored stools	
Low level	N/A	
After event, time until…		
Initial elevation	Hours	
Peak values	3–5 days	Assumes insult not removed
Normalization	Days	Assumes insult removed and no evolving damage
Causes of spurious results	Ascorbic acid	False elevation
Additional info	N/A	

Total Cholesterol

PARAMETER	DESCRIPTION	COMMENTS
Common reference range		
Adults	Desirable: <200 mg/dL	
	Borderline high: 200–239 mg/dL	
	High: ≥240 mg/dL	
Pediatrics		
(0–1 mo)	45–100 mg/dL	
(1–9 yr)	45–240 mg/dL	
(10–19 yr)	115–215 mg/dL	
Critical value	N/A	
Inherent activity	Not directly	Needed for cell wall, steroid, and bile acid production
Location		
Production	Liver and intestines	Ingested in diet
Storage	Fat	
Secretion/excretion	Excreted in bile	Some recycled to liver
Causes of abnormal levels		
High	Excess fat intake	
	Familial hypercholesterolemia	
Low	HMG-COA inhibitors, ezetimibe, niacin, fibric acids, bile acid sequestrants	Listed medications are commonly monitored
	Hyperthyroidism, malnutrition, anemia, liver disease	
Signs and symptoms		
High level	Atherosclerotic vascular disease	Angina, MI, CVA
Low level	N/A	
After event, time until…		
Initial elevation	Days to weeks	
Peak values	Days to weeks	
Normalization	Weeks to months	After change in diet or medication
Causes of spurious results	Prolonged tourniquet application	Increases 5% to 10%
Additional info	N/A	

Total Iron Binding Capacity (TIBC)

PARAMETER	DESCRIPTION	COMMENTS
Common reference range	250–410 mcg/dL	
Critical values	N/A	
Inherent activity	N/A	Measures the iron binding capacity of transferrin protein
Location	N/A	
Causes of abnormal levels		
High	Iron deficiency (GI/GU bleed, inadequate consumption, IBD, pica)	
Low	Infection, malignancy, inflammation, uremia, hemolytic anemia	
Signs and symptoms		
High level	Fatigue, pallor, tachycardia, numbness	
Low level	Fever, infectious symptoms, inflammation (depends on cause), jaundice	
After event, time until…	N/A	
Causes of spurious results	N/A	
Additional info	N/A	

Total Serum T3 (Triiodothyronine)

PARAMETER	DESCRIPTION	COMMENTS
Common reference range	78–195 ng/dL	Affected by TBG changes
Critical value	Not established	Extremely high or low values should be reported quickly
Inherent activity	Yes	Only free portion
Location		
Production/ storage	Thyroid gland; liver and kidneys	Bound mostly to thyroglobulin
Secretion/ excretion	From thyroid, liver and kidneys to blood	
Causes of abnormal levels		
High	T4/T3 supplements	Supplements and amiodarone routinely monitored
	Amiodarone, kelp, iodinated radiocontrast agents	
	Hyperthyroidism	Not a true cause but a reflection of a high level
Low	Propranolol, amiodarone, propylthiouracil, glucocorticoids	Amiodarone and propylthiouracil routinely monitored
	Hypothyroidism	Not a true cause but a reflection of a low level
Signs and symptoms		
High level	Nervousness, weight loss, heat intolerance, tachycardia, diaphoresis	Signs and symptoms of hyperthyroidism
Low level	Lethargy, constipation, dry skin, cold intolerance, confusion	Signs and symptoms of hypothyroidism
After event, time until…		
Initial elevation	Weeks to months	Increases within hours in acute T4 or T3 overdose
Peak values	Weeks to months	Increases within hours in acute T4 or T3 overdose
Normalization	Usually same time as onset	Assumes insult removed or effectively treated
Causes of spurious results	Increased or decreased TBG, Nonthyroidal illness	Increased or decreased TBG leads to falsely increased or decreased total serum T3 respectively
Additional info	N/A	

Total Serum T4 (Thyroxine)

PARAMETER	DESCRIPTION	COMMENTS
Common reference range		
Adults and children	4–12.5 mcg/dL	
Newborn	16–26 mcg/dL	
3–5 days	9–20 mcg/dL	
Critical value	Not established	Extremely high or low values should be reported quickly
Inherent activity	Only free portion	Total assumed to correlate with free T4 activity
Location		
Production	Thyroid gland	
Storage	Thyroid gland	Bound mostly to thyroglobulin
Secretion/ excretion	From thyroid to blood	33% converted to T3 outside thyroid
Causes of abnormal levels		
High	T4 supplements, hyperthyroidism	Levels commonly monitored with supplementation
Low	Hypothyroidism	
Signs and symptoms		
High level	Nervousness, weight loss, heat intolerance, tachycardia, diaphoresis	Signs and symptoms of hyperthyroidism
Low level	Lethargy, constipation, dry skin, cold intolerance, slow speech, confusion	Signs and symptoms of hypothyroidism
After event, time until…		
Initial elevation	Weeks to months	
Peak values	Weeks to months	Increases within hours in acute T4 overdose
Normalization	Same as onset	Assumes insult removed or effectively treated
Causes of spurious results	TBG abnormalities	Dependent on assay
Additional info	N/A	

Transferrin Saturation (TSAT)

PARAMETER	DESCRIPTION	COMMENTS
Common reference range	25% to 50%	<15% consistent with IDA (but limited specificity), >50% chronically is associated with iron overload
Critical values	N/A	
Inherent activity	N/A	Transferrin is the protein to which iron binds in the blood
Location	N/A	
Causes of abnormal levels		
High	Iron toxicity	Exogenous iron commonly initiated when TSAT<20%
Low	Iron deficiency, inflammation/infection/fever	
Signs and symptoms		
High level	Iron toxicity (CHF, cirrhosis, diabetes)	
Low level	Fatigue, pallor, tachycardia, numbness, fever, infectious symptoms, inflammation (depends on cause)	
After event, time until…	N/A	
Causes of spurious results	N/A	
Additional info	TSAT = serum iron/TIBC	

Tricyclic Antidepressant Levels

PARAMETER	DESCRIPTION	COMMENTS
Common reference range	Amitriptyline (A): combined A+N levels 120–250 mcg/L	A/N: midinterval level recommended
	Nortriptyline (N): 50–150 mcg/L	I/D: midinterval level recommended
	Imipramine (I): combined I+D levels 180–350 mcg/L	
	Desipramine (D): 115–250 mcg/L	
Critical values	A+N > 450 mcg/L	
	I+D > 500 mcg/L	
Inherent activity	Increase norepinephrine and serotonin neurotransmission	Also anticholinergic and alpha-1 antagonist properties
Location	N/A	
Causes of abnormal levels		
High	2D6 inhibitors	Levels not commonly monitored
Low	2D6 inducers	
Signs and symptoms		
High level	Anticholinergic effects, QRS prolongation, seizures, coma	QRS prolongation, seizures, coma occur at 5 x therapeutic levels
Low level	N/A	
After event, time until…		
Normalization	A/N: up to 11 days until steady state	
	I/D: up to 6 days until steady state	
Causes of spurious results	Carbamazepine may cause false positives with polyclonal antibody assay	
	Falsely low readings may occur in high alpha-1-acid glycoprotein (including cardiac and alcoholic patients)	
Additional info	Desipramine and nortriptyline are metabolites of imipramine and amitriptyline respectively	Concentrations of metabolite must be measured and added to concentration of parent drug to determine if level is therapeutic

Triglycerides

PARAMETER	DESCRIPTION	COMMENTS
Common reference range	Normal: <150 mg/dL	
	Borderline high: 150–199 mg/dL	
	High: 200–499 mg/dL	
	Very high: >500 mg/dL	
Critical value	>500 mg/dL	
Inherent activity	No	Needed for formation of other lipids and fatty acids
Location		
Production	Liver and intestines	
Storage	Fat	
Secretion/ excretion	Bile	
Causes of abnormal levels		
High	Amiodarone, atypical antipsychotics, beta-blockers, contraceptives (estrogen and progesterone), corticosteroids, cyclosporine, propofol, thiazide diuretics, sirolimus	Atypical antipsychotics routinely monitored
	Excess fat intake, excess carbohydrate intake, genetic defects, alcohol	
Low	Nicotinic acid, fibrates, omega-3 fatty acids, HMG-COA reductase inhibitors	Listed medications are commonly monitored
Signs and symptoms		
High level	Pancreatitis	
	Xanthomas	Levels >2000 mg/dL
	Lipemia retinalis	Levels >4000 mg/dL
Low level	None	
After event, time until…		
Initial elevation	Days to weeks	
Peak values	Days to weeks	
Normalization	Days to weeks	Assumes appropriate treatment
Causes of spurious results	Nonfasting sample	
Additional info	N/A	

Troponins I and T

PARAMETER	DESCRIPTION	COMMENTS
Common reference range	Troponin I: <0.5 ng/mL	Assay dependent
	Troponin T: <0.1 ng/mL	
Critical value	Troponin I: >1.5 ng/mL	Assay dependent
	Troponin T: >0.1 ng/mL	
Inherent activity	Yes	Regulates calcium-mediated interaction of actin and myosin
Location	Cardiac and skeletal muscle	Cardiac troponins I and T and skeletal muscle troponins I and T have different amino acid sequences
Causes of abnormal levels		
High	MI can cause mild elevations of TnI between 0.5–1.5 ng/mL; a "gray area" but indicates increased risk for a cardiac event	
	Other causes include cardiac surgery, coronary angioplasty, defibrillation, catheter ablation, resuscitation, myocarditis, heart failure, rejection of heart transplant, cardiac contusion, critical illness, PE, renal failure, chronic HD, rhabdomyolysis	
Low	N/A	No lower limit for normal
Signs and symptoms		
High level	Chest pain, N/V, diaphoresis	Abnormal HR and BP, anxiety, and confusion, depending on MI size, location, and duration
Low level	N/A	Does not cause signs and symptoms
After event, time until…		
Initial elevation	4–6 hr	Event: MI
		Time course studies of release needed
Peak values	12 hr to 2 days	
Normalization	5–14 days	
Causes of spurious results	N/A	
Additional info	For diagnosis of ACS, troponins should be checked after 6 hr from symptom onset; commonly evaluated whenever ACS is suspected	

Uric Acid (Serum)

PARAMETER	DESCRIPTION	COMMENTS
Common reference range		
Males >17 yr old	3.4–7 mg/dL	
Females >17 yr old	2.4– 6 mg/dL	
Critical value	>11 mg/dL	
Inherent activity	None	Metabolic end product of purines
Location		
Production	Liver	Produced from the degradation of dietary and endogenously synthesized purine compounds
Storage	Serum	
Secretion/excretion	Intestinal tract bacteria	
	Renal	
Causes of abnormal levels		
High	Low-dose ASA, pyrazinamide, nicotinic acid, ethambutol, ethanol, cyclosporine, acetazolamide, hydralazine, ethacrynic acid, furosemide, thiazide diuretics	Medications that may interfere with renal clearance of uric acid
	Methotrexate, nitrogen mustards, vincristine, azathioprine, 6-MP	Medications that increase production of uric acid; monitoring recommended for azathioprine and 6MP
	Leukemia, lymphoma, polycythemia, hemolytic anemia, sickle cell anemia, toxemia of pregnancy, psoriasis	Increased destruction of nucleoproteins
	Hypothyroidism, hypoparathyroidism, nephrogenic diabetes insipidus, Addison's disease	Endocrine abnormalities
Low	Allopurinol, probenecid, high-dose ASA (>3 g/day), high-dose vitamin C	
	Low protein diets, renal tubular defects, xanthine oxidase deficiency	
Signs and symptoms		
High level	Severe pain, redness, swelling	Gout related
	Other symptoms related to underlying cause	
Low level	N/A	
After event, time until…	N/A	
Causes of spurious results	Ascorbic acid >5 mg/dL, caffeine, theophylline, levodopa, methyldopa, propylthiouracil	False elevations
	Total bilirubin >10 mg/dL	False depression
Additional info	N/A	

Uric Acid (Urine)

PARAMETER	DESCRIPTION	COMMENTS
Common reference range	250–750 mg/24 hr	
Critical value	>1100 mg/24 hr	May necessitate initiation of prophylactic medication
Inherent activity	None	Metabolic end product of purines
Location		
Production	Liver	Produced from the degradation of dietary and endogenously synthesized purine compounds
Storage	Serum	
Secretion/ excretion	Intestinal tract bacteria	
	Renal	
Causes of abnormal levels		
High	Low-dose ASA, pyrazinamide, nicotinic acid, ethambutol, ethanol, cyclosporine, acetazolamide, hydralazine, ethacrynic acid, furosemide, thiazide diuretics	Medications that may interfere with renal clearance of uric acid; not commonly monitored unless symptoms
	Methotrexate, nitrogen mustards, vincristine, azathioprine, 6-MP	Medications that increase production of uric acid; monitoring recommended for azathioprine and 6MP
	Leukemia, lymphoma, polycythemia, hemolytic anemia, sickle cell anemia, toxemia of pregnancy, psoriasis	Increased destruction of nucleoproteins
	Hypothyroidism, hypoparathyroidism, nephrogenic diabetes insipidus, Addison's disease	Endocrine abnormalities
Low	Allopurinol, probenecid, high-dose ASA (>3 g/day), high-dose vitamin C	
	Low protein diets, renal tubular defects, xanthine oxidase deficiency	
Signs and symptoms		
High level	Severe pain, redness, swelling	Gout related
	Other symptoms related to underlying cause	
Low level	N/A	
After event, time until…	N/A	
Causes of spurious results	Ascorbic acid concentration >5 mg/dL, caffeine, theophylline, levodopa, methyldopa, propylthiouracil	False elevations
	Total bilirubin >10 mg/dL	False depression
Additional info	N/A	

Uridine Diphosphate Glucuronyl Transferase (UGT1A1)

PARAMETER	DESCRIPTION	COMMENTS
Common reference range	Presence of UGT1A1*1 genotype	Genotype testing
Critical value	Presence of UGT1A1 polymorphism	UGT1A1*28
Inherent activity	Yes	Enzyme responsible for the metabolism of SN-38 (a metabolite of irinotecan)
Location		
Production	N/A	
Storage	Serum	
Secretion/excretion	N/A	
Causes of abnormal levels		
High	Genetic polymorphism	
Low	N/A	
Signs and symptoms		
High level	Neutropenia	Related to elevated irinotecan levels
	GI toxicity	
Low level	N/A	
After event, time until...		
Initial elevation	N/A	
Peak values	N/A	
Normalization	N/A	
Causes of spurious results	N/A	
Additional info	FDA recommended a dose reduction of irinotecan in patients who have the UGT1A1*28 genotype	

Valproic Acid

PARAMETER	DESCRIPTION	COMMENTS
Common reference range	50–100 mg/L	Trough level recommended
	Some require levels up to 120 mg/L	Depakote ER® and Sprinkle® capsules formulations allow random levels
Critical values	Levels >175 mg/L associated with stupor/coma	
Inherent activity	Enhanced GABAergic neurotransmission	
Location	N/A	
Causes of abnormal levels		
High	Valproic acid	Levels are commonly monitored for efficacy and toxicity
Low	Low albumin states and drugs that displace valproic acid from albumin (e.g., salicylates) may cause falsely low total levels	
Signs and symptoms		
High level	>75 mg/L: ataxia, sedation, lethargy, fatigue	
	>100 mg/L: tremor	
	>175 mg/L: stupor, coma	
Low level	N/A	
After event, time until…		
Normalization	Steady state may require up to 5 days	
Causes of spurious results	Protein binding interactions, high serum concentrations	At higher concentrations, a greater percent of valproic acid is unbound and active
Additional info	N/A	

Vancomycin

PARAMETER	DESCRIPTION	COMMENTS
Common reference range	10–15 mg/L	Trough levels recommended
	15–20 mg/L, pneumonia, osteomyelitis, endocarditis, meningitis	
Critical values	N/A	
Inherent activity	Inhibits bacterial cell wall synthesis	
Location	N/A	
Causes of abnormal levels		
High	Renal impairment	Monitoring not necessary if normal renal function/ noncritically ill
Low	N/A	
Signs and symptoms		
High level	Red man syndrome (with >20 mg/min administration), nephrotoxicity (mostly with concurrent nephrotoxins), ototoxicity (associated with cumulative dose)	
Low level	N/A	
After event, time until…		
Normalization	Time until steady state depends on renal function	
Causes of spurious results	N/A	
Additional info	Levels not recommended for oral formulation due to lack of absorption	

Vitamin B12

PARAMETER	DESCRIPTION	COMMENTS
Common reference range	>200 pg/mL	Depends on assay
Critical values	N/A	
Inherent activity	Necessary for DNA and neurotransmitter synthesis, metabolism of homocysteine	
Location	Stored in liver	
Causes of abnormal levels		
High	Excess vitamin B12 administration	
Low	Colchicine, neomycin, para-aminosalicylic acid, nitrous oxide	It takes years to deplete stores of a normal liver
	Strict vegans, reduced gastric acidity (e.g., elderly, acid-suppressant therapies), IBD, ileal resection, gastrectomy	
Signs and symptoms		
High level	Restoration of B12 levels can cause hypokalemia and thrombocytosis	
Low level	Loss of appetite, abnormalities of taste/smell, paresthesias, macrocytic anemia, memory impairment	
After event, time until…		
Initial elevation	B12 levels quickly improve, many symptoms improve within a few days, Hgb begins to increase ~ a week	Event: B12 supplementation
Causes of spurious results	~5% of patients will have low B12 and a normal level due to assay interference by other cobamides	Due to this, methylmalonate and homocysteine levels are commonly ordered for diagnosis of B12 deficiency
Additional info	N/A	

White Blood Cell Count

PARAMETER	DESCRIPTION	COMMENTS
Common reference range		
Adults	$4.4–11.3 \times 10^3$ cells/mm³	
Newborns at birth	$9.0–30.0 \times 10^3$ cells/mm³	
2 wk old	$5.0–21.0 \times 10^3$ cells/mm³	
3 mo old	$6.0–18.0 \times 10^3$ cells/mm³	
0.5–6 yr old	$6.0–15.0 \times 10^3$ cells/mm³	
7–12 yr old	$4.5–13.5 \times 10^3$ cells/mm³	
Critical value	$>12 \times 10^3$ cells/mm³ (adult)	
	<500 cells/mm³	
Inherent activity	Yes	
Location		
Production	Bone marrow	
Storage	Bone marrow, serum	
Secretion/excretion	N/A	
Causes of abnormal levels		
High	Corticosteroids, epinephrine, lithium, G-CSF, GM-CSF	
	Acute/chronic bacterial infection	
	Trauma	
	MI	
	Leukemia	
Low	Antineoplastic cytotoxic agents, captopril, cephalosporins, chloramphenicol, clozapine, ganciclovir, methimazole, penicillins, phenothiazines, procainamide, ticlopidine, tricyclic antidepressants, vancomycin	
	Radiation exposure	
	Vitamin B12 or folate deficiency	
	Salmonellosis	
	Pertussis	
	Overwhelming bacterial infection	
Signs and symptoms		
High level	Related to underlying cause	
Low level	Related to underlying cause	

(continued)

White Blood Cell Count (Cont.)

After event, time until...	
Initial elevation	N/A
Peak values	N/A
Normalization	N/A
Causes of spurious results	N/A
Additional info	N/A

Zinc

PARAMETER	DESCRIPTION	COMMENTS
Common reference range	70–130 mcg/dL (10.7–19.9 μmol/L)	
Critical value	<70 mcg/dL (<10.7 μmol/L)	
Inherent activity	Yes	Enzyme constituent and cofactor, metabolism, tissue growth/repair, bone turnover, immune response, food intake control, spermatogenesis and gonadal maturation
Location		
Storage	Liver, pancreas, spleen, lungs, eyes (retina, iris, cornea, lens), prostate, skeletal muscle, bone, erythrocytes, neutrophils	60% to 62% in skeletal muscle, 20% to 28% in bone, 2% to 4% in liver
Secretion/excretion	Primarily in pancreatic and intestinal secretions; also lost dermally through sweat, hair and nail growth, and skin shedding	Only 2% lost in urine except in certain disease states
Causes of abnormal levels		
High	Zinc supplements, possibly during chronic TPN	Serum zinc concentrations not routinely monitored
Low	Low intake (infants), decreased absorption (acrodermatitis enteropathica), increased utilization (rapidly growing adolescents and menstruating, lactating, or pregnant women), increased loss (hyperzincuria)	
Signs and symptoms		
High level	Drowsiness, lethargy, N/V, diarrhea, increases in serum lipase and amylase concentrations	
Low level	Impaired immunity, pica, poor wound healing, impaired fetal development, decreased metabolism	
After event, time until…	N/A	
Causes of spurious results	Hemolyzed samples; 24-hr intrapatient variability	High zinc content in erythrocytes and neutrophils
Additional info	N/A	

Statistical Concepts Associated with Diagnosis

Negative post-test odds—when a negative result occurs, calculates the odds that it truly reflects absence of disease (takes pre-test odds and test predictive abilities into account).

Negative result likelihood ratio—the odds of a patient not having disease given a negative result.

Negative predictive value—the percent of patients without disease given a negative result.

Positive post-test odds—when a positive result occurs, calculates the odds that it truly reflects disease (takes pre-test odds and test predictive abilities into account).

Positive predictive value—the percent of patients with disease given a positive result.

Positive result likelihood ratio—the odds of a patient having disease given a positive result.

Pretest odds—similar to pretest probability except expressed as odds.

Pretest probability—the likelihood that a patient has the disease being assessed before the test is performed. For many disease states, there are calculations based on objective/subjective data that can estimate pretest probability.

Sensitivity—ability to identify positive results in patients with disease. The higher the sensitivity, the lower the chance of false-negative results. A sensitive test is needed to screen for diseases. Sensitivity = true positives/(true positives + false negatives).

Specificity—ability to identify negative results in patients without disease. The higher the specificity, the lower the chance of false-positive results. A specific test is needed to confirm a diagnosis. Specificity = true negatives/(false positives + true negatives).

	Disease Present	**Disease Absent**	
Test Positive	A	B	A + B
Test Negative	C	D	C + D
	A + C	B + D	A + B + C + D

Sensitivity	A/(A + C)
Specificity	D/(B + D)
Pretest Probability	(A + C)/(A + B + C + D)
Positive Predictive Value	A/(A + B)
Negative Predictive Value	D/(C + D)

(*continued*)

Likelihood Ratio (+)	(A/(A + C))/(1–(D/(B + D)))
Likelihood Ratio (–)	(1–(A/(A + C)))/(D/(B + D))
Pretest Odds	((A + C)/(A + B + C + D))/(1–((A + C)/(A + B + C + D))
Negative Post-test Odds	((A + C)/(A + B + C + D))/(1–((A + C)/(A + B + C + D))* (A/(A + C))/(1–(D/(B + D)))
Positive Post-test Odds	((A + C)/(A + B + C + D))/(1–((A + C)/(A + B + C + D))* (1–(A/(A + C)))/(D/(B + D))

General Information About Assay Modalities

Assay	Abbreviation	Analysis Time	Common Tests/Comments
Ion sensitive electrodes	ISE	6–18 min	Serum and urine electrolytes, simple and sensitive assay
Gas chromatography	GC	30 min	Toxicologic screens, organic acids, drug levels; one of the mainstays for drug detection; relies on differences in boiling points of analytes in sample
High-performance liquid chromatography	HPLC	30 min	Toxicologic screens, amino acids, drug levels; one of the mainstays for drug detection; relies on differences in solubility of analytes in sample
Enzyme-linked immunosorbent assay	ELISA	0.1–0.3 min	Serologic tests (e.g., antigens and antibodies); relies on immune-mediated reactions to improve sensitivity/specificity of assay
Enzyme-multiplied immunoassay	EMIT	0.1–0.3 min	General chemistries, enzymes, drug levels; relies on immune-mediated reactions to improve sensitivity/specificity of assay
Fluorescent polarization immunoassay	FPIA	0.1–0.2 min	Drug levels, general chemistries; relies on immune-mediated reactions to improve sensitivity/specificity of assay
Polymerase chain reaction	PCR	0.1–0.2 min	Microbiologic and virologic markers of organisms and genetic markers; amplifies DNA and RNA sequences to allow detection

Tubes for Blood Collection

Cap Color	Additive(s)	Laboratory Use and Comments
Brown	Sodium heparin	For lead determinations
Gold	Clot activator and gel for serum separation	For serum separation
Gray	Potassium oxalate/sodium fluoride Sodium fluoride Lithium iodoacetate Lithium iodoacetate/heparin Heparin sodium	For glucose, lactate, alcohol, and bicarbonate determinations; oxalate and heparin give plasma samples-without them, samples are serum; for lactate (on ice)
Green	Heparin sodium Lithium heparin Ammonium heparin	For plasma determinations in chemistry; used for arterial blood gasses, ammonia (on ice), and electrolytes
Lavender	Liquid potassium EDTA Freeze-dried sodium EDTA	For whole-blood hematology determinations
Light blue	0.105 M sodium citrate 3.2% 0.129 M sodium citrate 3.8%	For coagulation determinations on plasma; some tests require chilling
Light green	Lithium heparin and gel for plasma separation	Plasma separation tube for plasma determinations
Orange	Thrombin	For stat serum determinations in chemistry
Red	None	For serum determinations in chemistry, serology, and blood banking
Royal blue	Heparin sodium Sodium EDTA None	For trace element, toxicology, and nutrient determinations; not for chromium, manganese, aluminum and selenium
Yellow	Sodium polyanetholsulfonate (SPS) ACD Solution B of trisodium citrate	For blood culture specimen collections in microbiology; for blood banking and histocompatibility testing

Topic Index

Topic	Laboratory Value
Arterial Blood Gases and Acid-Base Balance	Anion gap
Arterial Blood Gases and Acid-Base Balance	Bicarbonate (HCO_3)/total CO_2 (venous)
Arterial Blood Gases and Acid-Base Balance	Ethylene glycol
Arterial Blood Gases and Acid-Base Balance	Lactate (lactic acid)
Arterial Blood Gases and Acid-Base Balance	Methanol
Arterial Blood Gases and Acid-Base Balance	O_2 saturation
Arterial Blood Gases and Acid-Base Balance	Partial pressure of arterial carbon dioxide ($PaCO_2$ or PCO_2)
Arterial Blood Gases and Acid-Base Balance	Partial pressure of arterial oxygen (PaO_2 or PO_2)
Arterial Blood Gases and Acid-Base Balance	pH (of arterial blood)
Cancers and Tumor Markers	Alpha-fetoprotein (AFp)
Cancers and Tumor Markers	BCR-ABL fusion gene
Cancers and Tumor Markers	Beta-2-microglobulin (B2M)
Cancers and Tumor Markers	CA 125 (cancer antigen 125)
Cancers and Tumor Markers	CA 15-3 (cancer antigen 15-3)
Cancers and Tumor Markers	CA 19-9 (cancer antigen 19-9)
Cancers and Tumor Markers	CA 27.29 (cancer antigen 27.29)
Cancers and Tumor Markers	Carcinoembryonic antigen (CEA)
Cancers and Tumor Markers	Estrogen and progesterone receptors
Cancers and Tumor Markers	Human chorionic gonadotropin (HCG)
Cancers and Tumor Markers	Human epidermal growth factor receptor 2 (HER-2)
Common Medical Disorders of Aging Males—Clinical and Laboratory Test Monitoring	PSA (prostate-specific antigen)
Common Medical Disorders of Aging Males—Clinical and Laboratory Test Monitoring	Testosterone
Electrolytes, Other Minerals, and Trace Elements	Calcium
Electrolytes, Other Minerals, and Trace Elements	Chloride
Electrolytes, Other Minerals, and Trace Elements	Chromium
Electrolytes, Other Minerals, and Trace Elements	Copper

Topic	Laboratory Value
Electrolytes, Other Minerals, and Trace Elements	Magnesium
Electrolytes, Other Minerals, and Trace Elements	Manganese
Electrolytes, Other Minerals, and Trace Elements	Phosphate
Electrolytes, Other Minerals, and Trace Elements	Potassium
Electrolytes, Other Minerals, and Trace Elements	Serum osmolality
Electrolytes, Other Minerals, and Trace Elements	Sodium
Electrolytes, Other Minerals, and Trace Elements	Zinc
Endocrine Disorders	C-peptide
Endocrine Disorders	Free T4 (thyroxine)
Endocrine Disorders	Fructosamine
Endocrine Disorders	Hemoglobin A1c
Endocrine Disorders	Plasma glucose
Endocrine Disorders	Thyroid stimulating hormone (TSH)
Endocrine Disorders	Total serum T3 (triiodothyronine)
Endocrine Disorders	Total serum T4 (thyroxine)
Hematology: Blood Coagulation Tests	Antifactor Xa activity
Hematology: Blood Coagulation Tests	Antiphospholipid antibodies
Hematology: Blood Coagulation Tests	Antithrombin
Hematology: Blood Coagulation Tests	aPTT (activated partial thromboplastin time)
Hematology: Blood Coagulation Tests	D-dimer
Hematology: Blood Coagulation Tests	Factor V Leiden
Hematology: Blood Coagulation Tests	Heparin-induced platelet antibodies
Hematology: Blood Coagulation Tests	INR/PT (international normalized ratio and prothrombin time)
Hematology: Blood Coagulation Tests	Platelet count
Hematology: Blood Coagulation Tests	Protein C & S
Hematology: Blood Coagulation Tests	Serotonin release assay (SRA)
Hematology: Red and White Blood Cell Tests	Coombs' test (direct)
Hematology: Red and White Blood Cell Tests	Ferritin
Hematology: Red and White Blood Cell Tests	Folate
Hematology: Red and White Blood Cell Tests	G6PD (glucose-6-phosphate dehydrogenase)

Topic	Laboratory Value
Hematology: Red and White Blood Cell Tests	Haptoglobin
Hematology: Red and White Blood Cell Tests	Hemoglobin (Hgb)/hematocrit (Hct)
Hematology: Red and White Blood Cell Tests	Homocysteine
Hematology: Red and White Blood Cell Tests	LDH (lactic acid dehydrogenase)
Hematology: Red and White Blood Cell Tests	Mean corpuscular hemoglobin concentration (MCHC)
Hematology: Red and White Blood Cell Tests	Mean corpuscular Hgb (MCH)
Hematology: Red and White Blood Cell Tests	Mean corpuscular volume
Hematology: Red and White Blood Cell Tests	Methylmalonate
Hematology: Red and White Blood Cell Tests	RBC distribution width (RDW)
Hematology: Red and White Blood Cell Tests	Red blood cells (RBC)
Hematology: Red and White Blood Cell Tests	Reticulocyte count
Hematology: Red and White Blood Cell Tests	Serum iron
Hematology: Red and White Blood Cell Tests	Total iron binding capacity (TIBC)
Hematology: Red and White Blood Cell Tests	Transferrin saturation (TSAT)
Hematology: Red and White Blood Cell Tests	Vitamin B12
Infectious Diseases	$1{\rightarrow}3$ β-D-glucan
Infectious Diseases	Band neutrophils
Infectious Diseases	Basophils
Infectious Diseases	CD4+ T lymphocyte count
Infectious Diseases	Eosinophils
Infectious Diseases	Galactomannan assay
Infectious Diseases	HIV antibody test
Infectious Diseases	HIV DNA PCR
Infectious Diseases	HIV RNA concentration (viral load)
Infectious Diseases	HIV Western blot
Infectious Diseases	HLA-B*5701
Infectious Diseases	Lymphocytes
Infectious Diseases	Mantoux test
Infectious Diseases	Monocytes
Infectious Diseases	Polymorphonuclear neutrophils

Topic	Laboratory Value
Liver and Gastroenterology Tests	Prealbumin
Liver and Gastroenterology Tests	Total bilirubin
Pharmacogenomics and Laboratory Tests	Thiopurine methyltransferase (TPMT)
Pharmacogenomics and Laboratory Tests	Uridine diphosphate glucuronyltransferase (UGT1a1)
Pulmonary Function and Related Tests	FEV_1 (forced expiratory volume in 1 sec)
Pulmonary Function and Related Tests	FEV_1/FVC
Pulmonary Function and Related Tests	PEFR (peak expiratory flow rate)
Rheumatic Diseases	Antinuclear antibodies (ANA)
Rheumatic Diseases	C3 and C4
Rheumatic Diseases	Complement hemolytic 50%
Rheumatic Diseases	C-reactive protein (CRP)
Rheumatic Diseases	Erythrocyte sedimentation rate (ESR)
Rheumatic Diseases	Rheumatoid factor
Rheumatic Diseases	Uric acid (serum)
Rheumatic Diseases	Uric acid (urine)
Substance Abuse and Toxicological Tests	Amphetamines and methamphetamines (urine drug screen)
Substance Abuse and Toxicological Tests	Barbiturates (urine drug screen)
Substance Abuse and Toxicological Tests	Benzodiazepines (urine drug screen)
Substance Abuse and Toxicological Tests	Benzoylecgonine (cocaine metabolite) (urine drug screen)
Substance Abuse and Toxicological Tests	Delta-9-tetrahydrocannabinol-9-carbozylic acid (THC) (urine drug screen)
Substance Abuse and Toxicological Tests	Lysergic acid diethylamide (LSD) (urine drug screen)
Substance Abuse and Toxicological Tests	Opiates (urine drug screen)
Substance Abuse and Toxicological Tests	Phencyclidine (PCP) (urine drug screen)
The Heart: Laboratory Tests and Diagnostic Procedures	B-type natriuretic peptide (BNP) & NT-proBNP
The Heart: Laboratory Tests and Diagnostic Procedures	CK-MB isoenzyme subforms (CK-MB1 and CK-MB2)
The Heart: Laboratory Tests and Diagnostic Procedures	CK-MB isoenzymes

Topic	Laboratory Value
The Heart: Laboratory Tests and Diagnostic Procedures	Creatine kinase (CK)
The Heart: Laboratory Tests and Diagnostic Procedures	Troponins I and T
The Kidneys	Adrenocorticotropic hormone (ACTH)
The Kidneys	Blood urea nitrogen (BUN)
The Kidneys	Cortisol (urine)
The Kidneys	Cosyntropin stimulation test
The Kidneys	Fractional excretion of sodium (FENa)
The Kidneys	Fractional excretion of urea (FEUrea)
The Kidneys	Serum creatinine (SCr)
Women's Health	Estradiol
Women's Health	FSH (follicle stimulating hormone)
Women's Health	LH (luteinizing hormone)
Women's Health	Progesterone
Women's Health	Prolactin

Index